Inflammatory Breast Cancer

Jaime G. de la Garza-Salazar
Abelardo Meneses-Garcia
Claudia Arce-Salinas
Editors

Inflammatory Breast Cancer

Springer

Editors
Jaime G. de la Garza-Salazar, M.D.
Department of Clinical Investigation
Instituto Nacional de
Cancerología-Mexico
Mexico City
Mexico

Claudia Arce-Salinas, M.D., M.Sc.
Department of Medical Oncology
Instituto Nacional de
Cancerologia-Mexico
Mexico City
Mexico

Abelardo Meneses-Garcia, Ph.D., M.D.
Department of Medical Direction
Instituto Nacional de
Cancerología-Mexico
Mexico City
Mexico

ISBN 978-0-85729-990-1 ISBN 978-0-85729-991-8 (eBook)
DOI 10.1007/978-0-85729-991-8
Springer London Heidelberg New York Dordrecht

Library of Congress Control Number: 2012948002

Printed on acid-free paper

Springer is part of Springer Science+Business Media (www.springer.com)

I dedicate this book to all breast cancer patients from the Instituto Nacional de Cancerologia-Mexico whose encouragement helped me keep working until we completed this book, thanks to all.

Dedicatoria

A todas las pacientes con cáncer de mama de nuestro Instituto Nacional de Cancerología-México motivo de inspiración clínica y de investigación.

Particularmente para mis primeras pacientes en 1970 y mis colegas oncólogos que creyeron y desearon junto conmigo romper un paradigma en el tratamiento del Carcinoma Inflamatorio de la Mama modelo de agresividad y mortalidad en el corto plazo.

A ellas con mi más profundo respeto y admiración.

Dr. Jaime G. de la Garza-Salazar.
Editor en Jefe

Preface

To write a book about inflammatory breast cancer (IBC) is something that I have had in mind for many years…

Why now? Well, there are a very good number of reports, articles, and symposiums about this pathology; all of the publications available at present are fragmented; and there are hundreds or thousands of articles associated with locally advanced breast cancer (LABC). I have invited different experts from the Instituto Nacional de Cancerologia-Mexico to investigate and review the most recent information on IBC regarding epidemiology, histopathology, clinical diagnosis, radiology and imaging, chemotherapy, radiotherapy, molecular biology, target therapy, and follow-up.

Major advances have been achieved over the past 42 years with respect to early diagnosis and immediate treatment with primary chemotherapy followed by surgery and radiotherapy. We are the pioneers in utilizing this different method of management (1970).

In a report from the MD Anderson Cancer Centre, A.M. González-Angulo and G. Hortobagyi conducted a study to evaluate whether the survival of women with IBC treated at our institution has improved over the past 30 years. The median follow-up was 5.8 years (range, 0.3–23.8 years). The median recurrence-free survival (RFS) duration was 2.3 years, and median overall survival (OS) time was 4.2 years. The conclusion: Data show that there has not been an important change in the prognosis of patients with IBC in the last 30 years. Clinical trials focusing on the management of this aggressive disease are warranted.

The history at our Institute in Mexico is that 42 years ago, the majority of patients with IBC, following treatment with surgery and radiotherapy, were dead 1 year after diagnosis. We demonstrated then that administering primary chemotherapy followed with radiotherapy and surgery showed good results. This 6-year experience with 18 patients was presented at the American Society of Clinical Oncology (ASCO) meeting in Denver, Colorado, in 1977.

At present and in our experience, there is no doubt that this method is indicated with anthracyclines as the central drug in any chemotherapy combination. Hope is sparked by the expectations of a future in which biological (target) therapies will improve complete responses as well as prolong the survival of persons suffering from IBC.

Mexico City, Mexico — Jaime G. de la Garza-Salazar

Acknowledgments

We would like to acknowledge the following people: Maggie Brunner (English translation and corrections), Sandra Garnica (secretarial work), Edmundo Alvarez (computer system advisor), and Daniel Dominguez (project manager).

Contents

Contributors

Lesvia Olivia Aguilar-Cortazar Department of Radiology, Instituto Nacional de Cancerologia-Mexico, Mexico City, DF, Mexico

Jose Luis Aguilar-Ponce, M.D. Department of Medical Oncology, Instituto Nacional de Cancerologia-Mexico, Mexico City, DF, Mexico

Claudia Arce-Salinas, M.D., M.Sc. Breast Tumor Department, Instituto Nacional de Cancerologia-Mexico (INCan), Mexico City, DF, Mexico

Department of Medical Oncology, Instituto Nacional de Cancerologia-Mexico, Mexico City, DF, Mexico

Oscar Gerardo Arrieta-Rodriguez, M.D. Department of Investigation, Instituto Nacional de Cancerologia-Mexico, Mexico City, DF, Mexico

Horacio Astudillo-de La Vega, M.D., M.Sc., Ph.D. Laboratory of Translational Research in Cancer, Oncology Hospital, National Medical Center "Siglo XXI", Instituto Mexicano del Seguro Social (IMSS), Mexico City, DF, Mexico

Juan Enrique Bargallo-Rocha, M.D. Breast Cancer Department, Instituto Nacional de Cancerologia-Mexico, Mexico City, DF, Mexico

Silvia Patricia Villarreal-Colin, M.D. Department of Medical Oncology, Instituto Nacional de Cancerologia-Mexico, Mexico City, DF, Mexico

Breast Tumor Department, Instituto Nacional de Cancerología-México (INCan), Mexico City, DF, Mexico

Roberto Alejandro Cruz-Morales Department of Radiology, Instituto Nacional de Cancerologia-Mexico, Mexico City, DF, Mexico

Jaime Ignacio Garcia-Gomez Department of Radiology, Instituto Nacional de Cancerologia-Mexico, Mexico City, DF, Mexico

Martin Granados-Garcia Department of Surgical Oncology, Instituto Nacional de Cancerologia-Mexico, Mexico City, DF, Mexico

Jaime G. de la Garza-Salazar, M.D. Department of Clinical Investigation, Instituto Nacional de Cancerologia-Mexico, Mexico City, DF, Mexico

Angel Herrera-Gomez, M.D. Department of Surgical Oncology, Instituto Nacional de Cancerologia-Mexico, Mexico City, DF, Mexico

Roque Alberto Guadarrama-Fleites, M.D. Department of Radiation Oncology, Instituto Nacional de Cancerologia-Mexico, Mexico City, DF, Mexico

Luis Alonso Herrera-Montalvo, Ph.D. Department of Biomedic Research in Cancer, Instituto Nacional de Cancerologia-Mexico, Mexico City, DF, Mexico

Paula Juarez-Sanchez, M.D. Department of Pathology, Instituto Nacional de Cancerologia-Mexico (INCan), Ssa, Mexico City, DF, Mexico

David F. Cantu-de Leon, Ph.D. Gynecologic Tumors Department, Instituto Nacional de Cancerologia-Mexico, Mexico City, DF, Mexico

Clinical Research Department, Instituto Nacional de Cancerologia-Mexico, Mexico City, DF, Mexico

Horacio Noe Lopez-Basave, M.S. Department of Oncological Surgery, Instituto Nacional de Cancerologia-Mexico, Mexico City, DF, Mexico

Hector Aquiles Maldonado-Martinez, M.D., Ph.D. Department of Pathology, Instituto Nacional de Cancerologia-Mexico, Mexico City, DF, Mexico

Fernando Lara-Medina, M.D. Department of Medical Oncology, Instituto Nacional de Cancerologia-Mexico, Mexico City, DF, Mexico

Abelardo Meneses-Garcia, M.D., Ph.D. Department of Medical Direction, Instituto Nacional de Cancerologia-Mexico, Mexico City, DF, Mexico

Alejandro Mohar-Betancourt, M.D., Ph.D. Department of General Direction, Instituto Nacional de Cancerología, Mexico City, DF, Mexico

Unit of Biomedical Research in Cancer, Instituto Nacional de Cancerología (INCan)

Flavia Morales-Vasquez, M.D., M.S. Department of Medical Oncology, Instituto Nacional de Cancerologia-Mexico, Mexico City, DF, Mexico

Aida Mota-Garcia, M.D. Department of Radiation Oncology, Instituto Nacional de Cancerologia-Mexico, Mexico City, DF, Mexico

Cecilia Magdalena Pavon-Hernandez Department of Radiology, Instituto Nacional de Cancerologia-Mexico, Mexico City, DF, Mexico

Martha Patricia Perez-Badillo Department of Radiology, Instituto Nacional de Cancerologia-Mexico, Mexico City, DF, Mexico

Victor Manuel Perez-Sanchez, M.D. Department of Pathology, Instituto Nacional de Cancerologia-Mexico, Mexico City, DF, Mexico

Irma Perez-Zuñiga Department of Radiology, Instituto Nacional de Cancerologia-Mexico, Mexico City, DF, Mexico

Maria Teresa Ramirez-Ugalde, M.D. Breast Tumor Department, Instituto Nacional de Cancerologia-Mexico, Mexico City, DF, Mexico

Nancy Reynoso-Noveron Department of Breast Tumors, Instituto Nacional de Cancerología, Mexico City, DF, Mexico

Universidad Nacional Autónoma de México (UNAM), Mexico City, DF, Mexico

Erika Ruiz-Garcia Translational Research in Cancer, Instituto Nacional de Cancerologia-Mexico, Mexico City, DF, Mexico

Juan Alberto Serrano-Olvera, M.D. Clinical Research Department, Instituto Nacional de Cancerologia-Mexico, Mexico City, DF, Mexico

Robin R. Shaw-Dulin, M.D. Breast Tumor Department, Instituto Nacional de Cancerologia-Mexico, Mexico City, DF, Mexico

Diana Vanesa Toledano-Cuevas, M.D. Department of Radiation Oncology, Instituto Nacional de Cancerologia-Mexico, Mexico City, DF, Mexico

Yolanda Villaseñor-Navarro Department of Radiology, Instituto Nacional de Cancerologia-Mexico, Mexico City, DF, Mexico

1 Introduction

Jaime G. de la Garza-Salazar
and Paula Juarez-Sanchez

Introduction

Inflammatory breast carcinoma (IBC) is the most aggressive manifestation of primary breast cancer [1].

The clinical presentation of IBC was first described in 1817 by Sir Charles Bell (Fig. 1.1) as "a purple color on the skin above the tumor accompanied by shooting pains."

Clinical presentation consisted of rapid onset and swelling of the skin [1]. Diagnostic criteria were established by Haagensen [2] and included diffuse erythema, edema involving more than two-thirds of the breast, *peau d'orange*, tenderness, induration, warmth, enlargement, and diffuseness of the tumor on palpation (Fig. 1.2). These symptoms usually progress rapidly, with axillary node involvement.

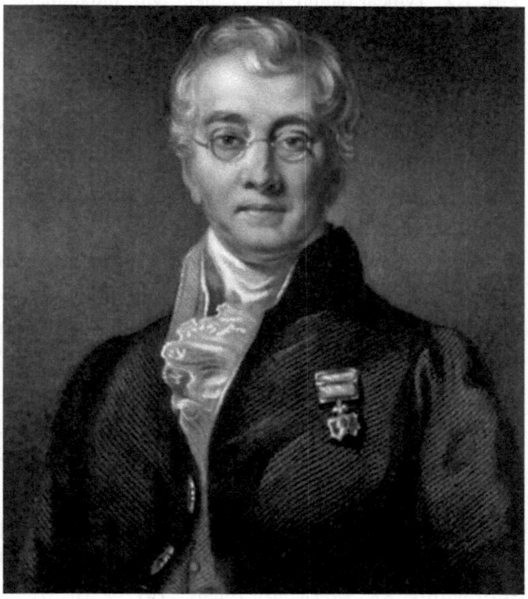

Fig. 1.1 Sir Charles Bell

IBC is a relatively rare entity in the USA, with an incidence of 1–6 %; however, its incidence varies according to its definition. Thus, when IBC is based on clinical and pathology findings, the incidence is lower (1–1.3 %) [3]; according to Surveillance, Epidemiology, and End Results (SEER), this is 2.0/100,000 person-years, in contrast with North Africa (Egypt and Tunisia), with a higher prevalence (10 %) [4].

Despite the high incidence of IBC in Africa, the latter has changed over time. In the decade of the 1970s, the prevalence of IBC was 70 % and

J.G. de la Garza-Salazar, M.D. (✉)
Department of Clinical Investigation,
Instituto Nacional de Cancerologia-Mexico,
Ave. San Fernando 22, Tlalpan, Mexico City,
DF 14080, Mexico
e-mail: jdelagarza1@prodigy.net.mx

P. Juarez-Sanchez, M.D.
Department of Pathology, Instituto Nacional de
Cancerologia-Mexico (INCan), Ssa,
Mexico City, DF, Mexico
e-mail: cendifarma2006@yahoo.com.mx

J.G. de la Garza-Salazar et al. (eds.), *Inflammatory Breast Cancer*,
DOI 10.1007/978-0-85729-991-8_1, © Springer-Verlag London 2013

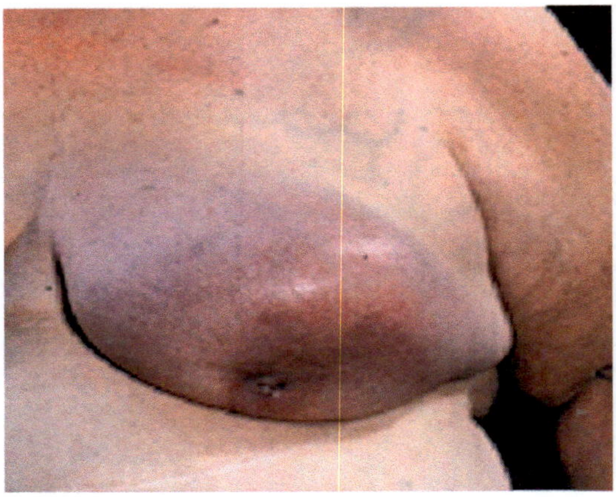

Fig. 1.2 Typical picture of a patient with inflammatory breast cancer

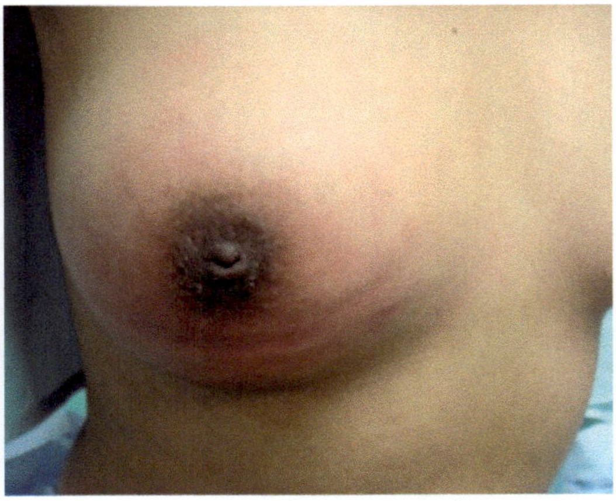

Fig. 1.3 Mastitis

has recently been reported as <10 %. This change has been attributed to more stringent definition criteria and also to improvement in socioeconomic levels [5].

At the Instituto Nacional de Cancerología (INCan) in Mexico City, among the 1,606 new cases of breast cancer seen at our institution between January 2006 and December 2008, IBC represented 5.1 % (n=82) of all cases.

Median age at diagnosis was 53 years (range, 23–85 years), and the majority of these cases are in postmenopausal status (59 %).

Invasive ductal carcinoma was the most common histological type at diagnosis and represents 88 % of all cases; 60 % of these are poorly differentiated, with lymphovascular invasion present in 18 %. According to the immunohistochemistry pattern, the tumor was classified as triple negative in 30.5 % (25 cases), as human epidermal growth factor receptor (HER)-positive immunohistochemistry [IHC] 3+ or fluorescence in situ hybridization [FISH] in 25.6 % (21), and as estrogen receptor (ER)-positive in 48.8 % (40). The clinical characteristics of IBC have been defined since 1953 by Haagensen. Currently, the American Joint Committee on Cancer (AJCC) defined IBC as "a clinic-pathological entity characterized by diffuse erythema and edema of the breast, often without an underlying palpable mass" [6].

Recently, a group of experts in IBC mentioned the diagnostic criteria, based in clinic and pathologic findings, and these are listed as follows [7]: (a) history of rapid onset of breast erythema, edema, and/or *peau d'orange*, and/or warm breast, with or without an underlying palpable mass; (b) history of flattening, crusting, or retraction of the nipple may be present; (c) patients may have a history of being diagnosed with mastitis and of not responding to at least 1 week of antibiotics; (d) duration of history of no more than 6 months; (e) clinical examination revealing erythema occupying at least one-third of the breast; (f) clinical examination may reveal underlying palpable mass with or without palpable locoregional lymph nodes with or without nipple abnormalities; (g) pathological confirmation of invasive carcinoma from a core biopsy of the breast; and (h) recommendation for obtaining an adequate skin punch biopsy to possibly document dermal lymphovascular tumor emboli. IBC is characterized by a minimal in situ component or a lack thereof. It is very important to possess a differential diagnosis; the most frequent of these comprise mastitis and abscess (Figs. 1.3 and 1.4).

There is often an extensive component of intraparenchymal lymphovascular tumor emboli. The IBC growth pattern is less compact than that of non-IBC (leaving more available space for migration of cancer cells) with large tumor-free

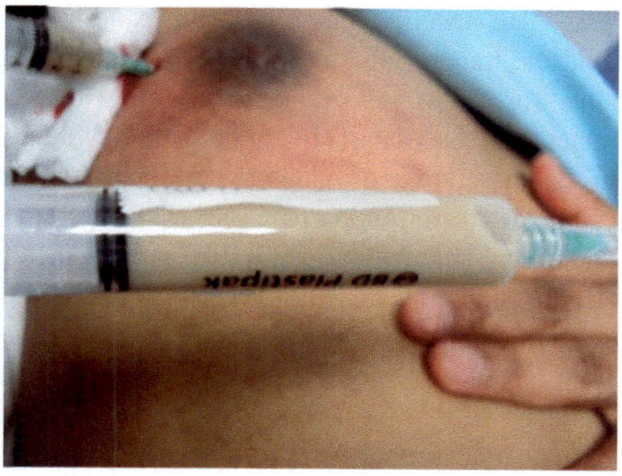

Fig. 1.4 Breast abscess

skip areas and small areas of invasive carcinoma, sometimes still surrounding vascular emboli.

The inflammatory skin changes of a breast afflicted with IBC represent the presence of dermal lymphatic invasion (DLI), a state in which dilated dermal lymphovascular spaces are filled with tumor emboli that are often retracted away from the surrounding endothelial lining [8]. Considered a histological hallmark of IBC, DLI subsequently leads to lymphatic obstruction and is ultimately responsible for the highly metastatic potential. DLI is identified in <75 % of patients with IBC, indicating that it is not an absolute requirement for diagnosis of IBC.

IBC is also characterized by the presence of molecular aggressive-disease markers, including high S-phase, aneuploidy, absent of ER expression, and high expression of p53 and HER2 [9].

Aziz et al. [10] compared the expression levels of several prognostic markers, including p53 in 40 IBC from 40 matched patients with non-IBC; the author shows that 70 % of inflammatory tumors have expression of p53 versus 48 % in the control group ($p=0.0238$). Other authors [11] have found a process of nuclear exclusion and cytoplasm sequestration as the predominant mechanism of protein function inactivation. The process of p53 inactivation by nuclear exclusion phenomenon has been found in 37 % of IBC and in approximately 95 % of undifferentiated neuroblastomas [12]. Further studies have clarified that the formation of cytoplasm aggregates is mediated by the C-terminal domain of p53 and results in high molecular weight complexes with half-lives of about 6 h.

The functions of Mdm2 and phosphatase and tensin homolog (PTEN) are thought to be critical to the regulation of p53 function. In fact, the level of p53 activity is regulated in part by the Mdm2 oncoprotein. Mdm2 shuttling from the cytoplasm to the nucleus promotes p53 protein degradation through the ubiquitin-dependent proteasome pathway. PTEN has been shown to inhibit the phosphatidylinositol 3-kinase/Akt signal that regulates Mdm2 translocation into the nucleus, resulting in persistent p53 activation [13]. PTEN is a tumor-suppressor gene localized at chromosome 10q23 that regulates cell migration, growth, and survival by dephosphorylating phosphatidylinositol 3-kinase second messengers and signaling phosphoproteins. Through this mechanism, PTEN also inhibits the nuclear entry of Mdm2, causing degradation by the proteasome and increasing the cellular content of p53. Loss of PTEN has been found in invasive breast cancer and has been associated with poor prognosis [14]. Cadherins are transmembranal components that play crucial roles in epithelial morphogenesis and that mediate intercellular adhesion [15].

These receptors bind catenins and are involved in signal transduction pathways that regulate cell growth and apoptosis. Epithelial cadherin (E-cadherin) is a potent tumor suppressor in breast cancer, and loss of E-cadherin expression has been found to correlate with poor prognosis [16]. Overexpression of E-cadherin has been described as characteristic of IBC; this biological characteristic explains the presence of diffuse lymphovascular tumor emboli and the lack of endothelial adherence of the cells constituting it [17].

Recent studies have indicated that interactions between chemokine receptors in breast cancer cells and their ligand in host organs play a role in malignant dissemination and progression [18]. The CXCR4 ligand CXCL12/SDF-1a is expressed in liver, bone marrow, lung, and lymph nodes, whereas the CCR7 ligand CCL21 is highly expressed in lymph nodes of patients with breast cancer. CXCR4 has been identified as a key mediator in neoangiogenesis; its effect is mediated by upregulating vascular endothelial growth factor (VEGF) [19]. Similarly, VEGF has been shown to increase CXCR4 expression, forming a positive feedback mechanism to promote angiogenesis [20].

Moreover, we recently showed cross-talk between CXCR4 and HER2-*neu*/epidermal growth factor receptor (EGFR) via HER2-*neu* and EGFR transactivation by the SDF-1a–CXCR4 axis [21]. CCR7 has been reported to play a key role in T-cell differentiation, and its presence on the cell surface divides memory T-cells into two subsets: effector memory (CCR7−) and central memory (CCR7+) T-cells, which possess different immune functions in secondary immune responses [22]. CCR7 has also been associated with an increased propensity for metastatic spread to lymph nodes.

A retrospective [23] study of 44 cases of IBC shows that 40.9 % of all participants had positive CXCR4, 22.7 % had positive CCR7, 47.7 % had positive HER2, and 30 % had EGFR positivity; this expression was associated with 5-year overall survival, which was 24.8 % for CXCR4-positive versus 42.3 % for CXCR4-negative and 20 % for CCR7-positive versus 41.9 % for CCR/7-negative patients, without statistical significance.

Several studies have demonstrated the high prevalence of HER2 expression. Parton et al. [24] reported the prevalence of HER2 of 52 % in 49 new cases. Perhaps this high expression, at present not associated with poor prognosis due to the introduction of trastuzumab in the treatment of breast cancer [25]. Cancers have been conceptualized as over-healing wounds or "wounds that do not heal," and wound repair-reflective gene expression signatures have demonstrated value as predictors of breast cancer survival. The in vivo wound response signature is highly prognostic of breast cancer survival [26].

IBC is characterized by a distinct gene expression signature compared with non-IBC [27]. This IBC-specific gene expression pattern may hold the fingerprints of the mechanisms responsible for the aggressive behavior and elevated metastatic potential of IBC tumor cells. Evidence in this direction is provided by the identification of nuclear factor-kappa beta (NF-κB) hyperactivation and augmented insulin-like growth factor (ILGF) signaling in IBC through genome-wide gene expression profiling. Both concepts have been linked with breast cancer metastasis. It has been shown that NF-κB activation mediates the cellular transformation, proliferation, invasion, angiogenesis, and metastasis of cancer. The ILGF pathway mediates cell motility through Rho GTPases via the phosphatidylinositol 3-kinase system, leading to an increased invasive and metastatic potential in breast cancer. Thus, analysis of the RNA obtained from 17 IBC and 40 non-IBC samples indicates that classification according to the IBC signature is significantly ($p < 0.05$) associated with cell-of-origin subtypes, the wound-healing response, the invasive gene signature, the genomic grade index, the fibroblastic neoplasm signature, and the 70-gene prognostic signature [26].

Treatment of IBC must be primary systemic chemotherapy as first line of treatment with the aim of downstaging the tumor to allow for definitive surgery. In 1970, 40 years ago, all of our patients with IBC at the Oncology Hospital in Mexico City, at 12 months post-diagnosis, were dead regardless of the treatment received (surgery, radiotherapy, chemotherapy, hormonal ablation, etc.). We initiated in Mexico, and probably and to our knowledge in the world, a new and different management of inflammatory breast cancer: primary treatment with chemotherapy, 5-fluorouracil 10 mg/kg intravenous bolus daily for 5 days, then weekly for 2 months, followed by radiotherapy and surgery according to the response. In 1977, we presented our results at the American Society of Clinical Oncology (ASCO) meeting at Denver, Colorado (Abstract C-32), of a 6-year follow-up.

First patient treated in Mexico with primary chemotherapy in 1970 (Figs. 1.5 and 1.6)

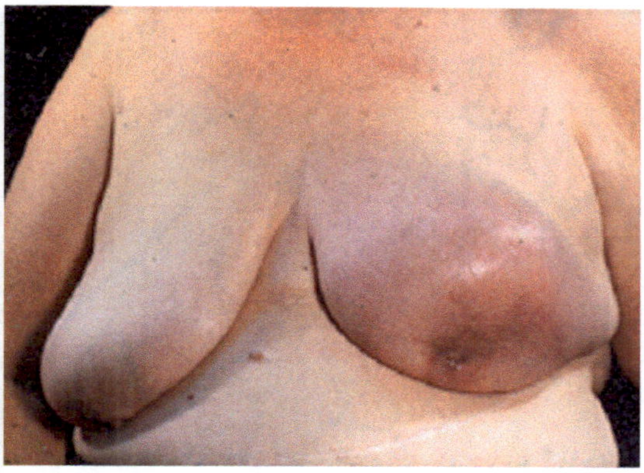

Fig. 1.5 First patient treated with primary chemotherapy in Mexico

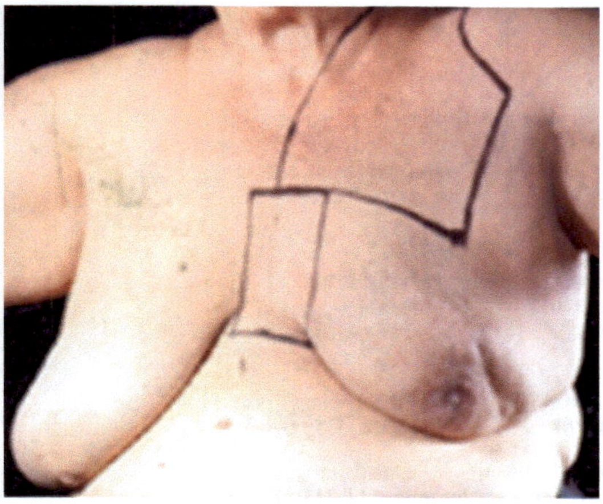

Fig. 1.6 Three months after primary chemotherapy with 5-fluorouracil

The first publication in Mexico reporting on 18 patients, 1977 (at 6 years of experience) (Figs. 1.7 and 1.8)

Authors of the 1977 publication at ASCO (Figs. 1.9, 1.10 and 1.11)

To our knowledge, there are no data from large randomized clinical trials that consider an optimal chemotherapeutic regimen specifically for women with IBC. The largest study considering 178 women with IBC who all received an anthracycline-based regimen followed by local therapy reported 5- and 10-year survival rates of 40 and 33 %, respectively [28]. Incorporation of taxanes has also shown to be associated with higher pathologic complete response (pCR) rates and better survival outcomes [29, 30]. Currently, there are no data to support the use of additional adjuvant chemotherapies in patients with residual disease.

Although the results of studies contemplating the use of high-dose chemotherapy among women with IBC have been encouraging, this treatment modality continues to be considered investigational and is not recommended outside the confines of a clinical trial [31, 32].

The Expert Panel strongly recommends the administration of trastuzumab to women with HER2-positive disease, with studies indicating that its addition to primary systemic chemotherapy is associated with higher pCR rates [7]. A recent prospective study that randomized women with locally advanced breast cancers, including those with IBC, to anthracycline-based chemotherapy with or without 1 year of trastuzumab (preoperative followed by adjuvant) demonstrated that the addition of trastuzumab significantly improved pCR rates (38 vs. 19 %; $p=0.001$) and event-free survival (3-year event-free survival, 71 vs. 56 %; HR 0.59; $p=0.013$) [33].

Recently, the IBC Panel of Experts recommended that a minimum of six cycles of preoperative treatment be administered over a 4–6-month course prior to proceeding to definitive surgery [7].

It is recommended that patients with IBC who undergo a modified radical mastectomy receive postmastectomy radiation therapy. The recommendation comprises radiation therapy including supraclavicular regions and internal mammary lymph nodes. It is also recommended that the cumulative radiation dose be escalated to 66 Gy in the subset of women aged <45 years who have close or positive surgical margins, four or more positive lymph nodes following preoperative systemic treatment, or who have demonstrated a poor response to preoperative systemic treatment [34].

The photograph is of a 65-year-old female diagnosed with inflammatory breast cancer on January 28, 2009. Adenocarcinoma, HER2/negative, and ER-PR negative (triple negative) 5-fluorouracil, adriamycin, cyclophosphamide

CIRUGIA
Y CIRUJANOS

Nº 6 TOMO XLV CIRUGIA Y CIRUJANOS

Organo oficial de la
Academia Mexicana de Cirugía

Contenido

Tomo XLV - No. 6 - Nov.-Dic., 1977
Publicación bimestral
(Cirug. y Cirujan.)

Fig. 1.7 First publication in Mexico 1977

Cáncer inflamatorio de la glándula mamaria. Experiencia de seis años con QT-RT-QT

Jaime G. de la Garza Salazar*

Se presentan dieciocho casos con diagnóstico clínico de carcinoma inflamatorio de la glándula mamaria, todos diagnosticados histológicamente como malignos; sólo en nueve de ellos se pudo confirmar el diagnóstico de permeación linfática debido a que en el resto se practicó biopsia por punción. Cuatro casos habían recibido tratamiento antineoplásico previo, quirúrgico o radioterápico; ninguna enferma fue tratada con hormonoterapia ablativa o aditiva; en forma inicial todas las enfermas recibieron 5-fluorouracilo por vía intravenosa rápida, sin diluciones, 10 mg. por kilogramo de peso, por cinco días, y posteriormente dosis semanal de 12 mg. por kilogramo, por un periodo mínimo de dos meses; se continuó después con irradiaciones, recibiendo ciclo mamario completo y variando las dosis entre 2 000 y 8 000 rads.

La toxicidad a la quimioterapia se observó en la esfera gastrointestinal sin ninguna consecuencia, en porcentajes variables; al suspender el fármaco durante un periodo de ocho días se recuperó el enfermo.

Desde el punto de vista hematológico se presentó, en un 44 por ciento, leucopenia de 3 000 a 4 000 leucocitos por mm³ y 16 por ciento de 2 000 leucocitos por mm³, sin llegar a considerarse un problema. Todas estas cifras se recuperaron al suspender la quimioterapia; la toxicidad a la radioterapia fue mínima, sólo se presentaron algunos casos de dermatitis que fueron fácilmente manejados.

Se comunican seis excelentes respuestas, diez buenas y dos malas. A seis años de iniciado este programa existen cuatro casos vivos, dos de los cuales están sin evidencia clínica de actividad tumoral a 63 y 48 meses; otras dos pacientes a 25 y 38 meses con actividad tumoral.

Dos de las enfermas con mala respuesta fallecieron a los cuatro y ocho meses de haber iniciado la quimioterapia.

Consideramos que la quimioterapia-radioterapia-quimioterapia (QT-RT-QT) es el método ideal para el manejo del cáncer inflamatorio de la mama y que una futura combinación será: adriamicina-ciclofosfamida y 5-fluorouracilo, seguida de ciclo mamario con radioterapia y posteriormente continuar con la quimioterapia durante un periodo de dos años.

El manejo hormonal debe ser de acuerdo a cada caso en particular.

Los resultados de esta diferente modalidad terapéutica brindan un 33.3 por ciento a las respuestas excelentes, con un tiempo de sobrevida de 39.3 meses, y a las buenas respuestas de un 55.5 por ciento y 20.6 meses promedio de sobrevida para un promedio global de 25.2 meses.

* Del Servicio de Quimioterapia del Hospital de Oncología, Centro Médico Nacional, Instituto Mexicano del Seguro Social.

351

Fig. 1.8 First publication in Mexico 1977

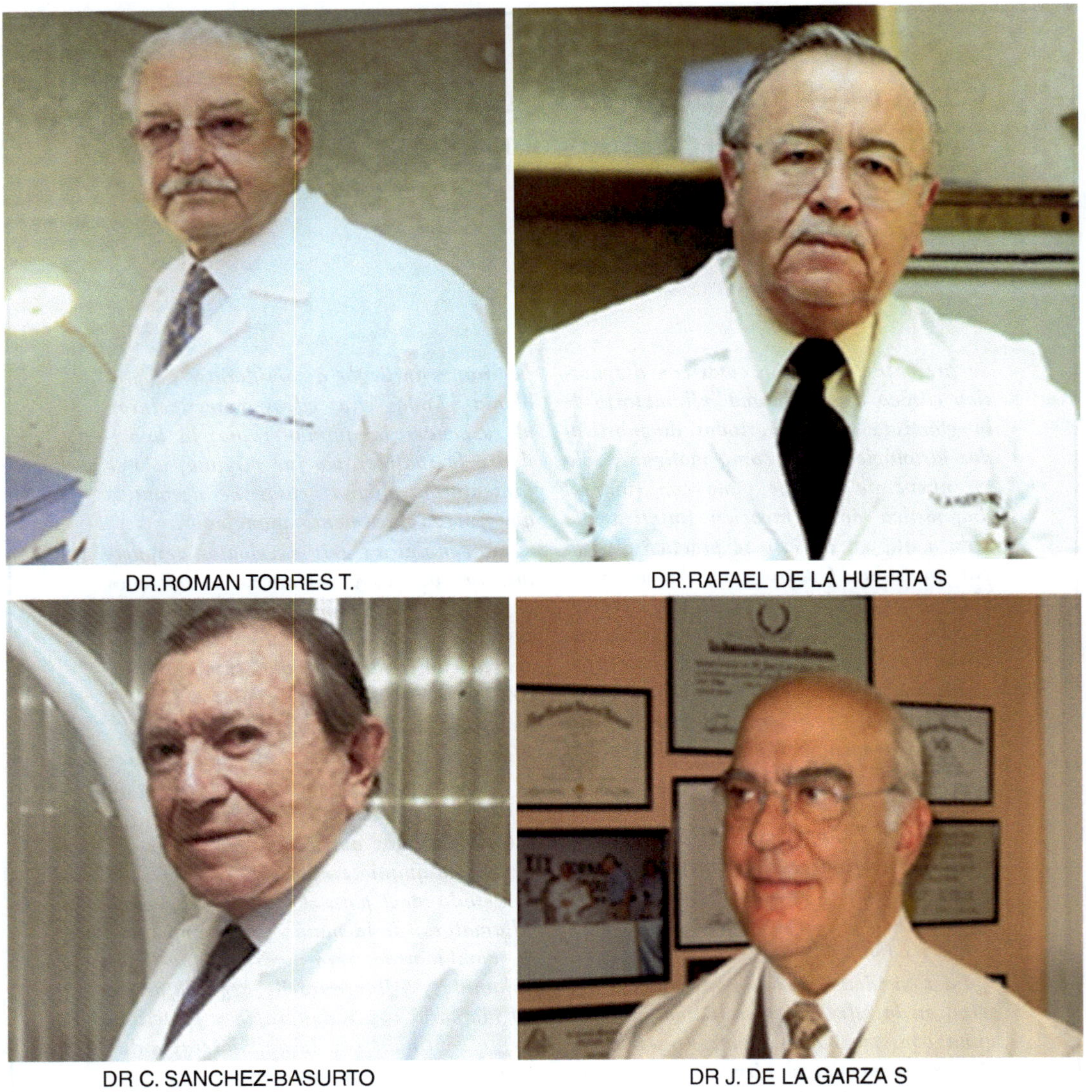

Fig. 1.9 Authors of the different management of IBC 1970

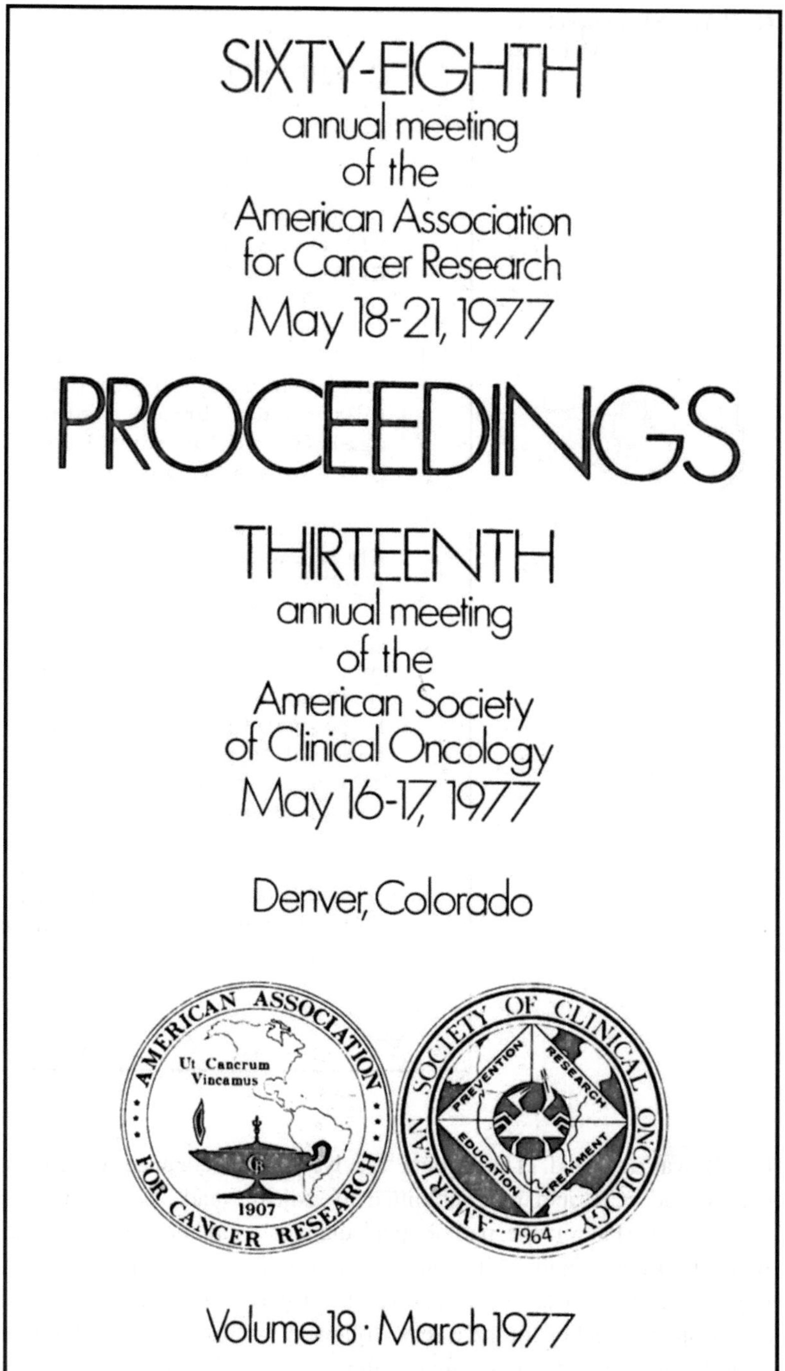

SIXTY-EIGHTH
annual meeting
of the
American Association
for Cancer Research
May 18-21, 1977

PROCEEDINGS

THIRTEENTH
annual meeting
of the
American Society
of Clinical Oncology
May 16-17, 1977

Denver, Colorado

Volume 18 · March 1977

Fig. 1.10 Publication of the Abstract C-32 ASCO, Denver 1977

C-32 DIFFERENT MANAGEMENT OF INFLAM MATORY BREAST CARCINOMA (CHEMO-RX-CHEMO) EXPERIENCE IN 18 CASES DURING A 6 YEARS PERIOD (1970-1976). Jaime G. de la Garza, Rafael de la Huerta, Román Torres and C. Sánchez B. H.ONCOLOGIA IMSS and Hosp. "20 de Noviembre" ISSSTE, Mexico City. Eighteen pts with Inflammatory breast carcino ma were initially treated for 2 mos. with 5FU Followed by radical radiation therapy and subse quently 2yrs of chemotherapy, single and com bined was used. In our Institution since 1970 Inflammatory breast carcinoma has been man aged with 5FU 10 mg x kg x 5 days IV push fol lowed by weekly dose (12 mg x kg x wk) for an average of 2 mos. period, this was followed by radical radiation therapy (supraclavicular ax illary and internal mammary fields 4000-6000 rads) followed by return to chemotherapy. Af ter 6 yrs (72 mos) of the initiation of this study we have had complete responses in 6 pts. with median survival of 39.3 mos. partial responses in 10 pts with median survival of 20.6 mos.; on ly two patients did not respond. At the present time only 4 patients are alive at 63, 48, 38 and 25 mos. 2 patients are disease free (63 and 48 mos.) Before the initiation of this study in our Hospitals the median survival rate for inflam matory breast carcinoma was 10 mos., there fore this new Modality has proven to be success full in the management of Inflammatory breast carcinoma.

PROCEEDINGS OF AACR AND ASCO

Fig. 1.11 Publication of the Abstract C-32 ASCO, Denver 1977

(FAC) was initiated. The patient received six cycles, had cCR, and was submitted to radical mastectomy (Patey); the pathological diagnosis was microscopic, and malignant cells and axillary lymph nodes were negative; paclitaxel was administered weekly for 12 weeks, followed by radiotherapy (linear accelerator). After 3 years without adjuvant therapy, the patient is disease-free and enjoys an excellent quality of life (QOL) (Figs. 1.12, 1.13 and 1.14).

To date, the treatment sequence has not been elucidated; a retrospective study was carried out to determine whether mastectomy use, chemotherapy intensity, or the treatment sequence of chemotherapy, radiation therapy, and mastectomy has improved the outcome demonstrated in 485 patients that mastectomy in conjunction with chemo- and radiation therapy enhances locoregional control regardless of the sequence. Moreover, chemotherapy improves breast cancer survival [35].

It is recommended that patients with hormone receptor-positive IBC receive a minimum of 5 years of hormone therapy with either tamoxifen or an aromatase inhibitor depending on their menopausal status. There are no current data that indicate the optimal duration of trastuzumab specifically among women with IBC. However,

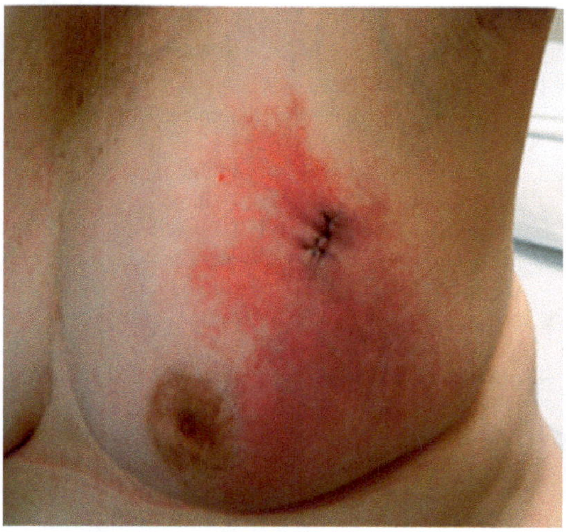

Fig. 1.12 Patient, with IBC triple negative, treated with 5-fluorouracil, adriamycin, cyclophosphamide (*FAC*) (six cycles) followed by radical surgery + paclitaxel (weekly × 12 weeks) followed by radiotherapy

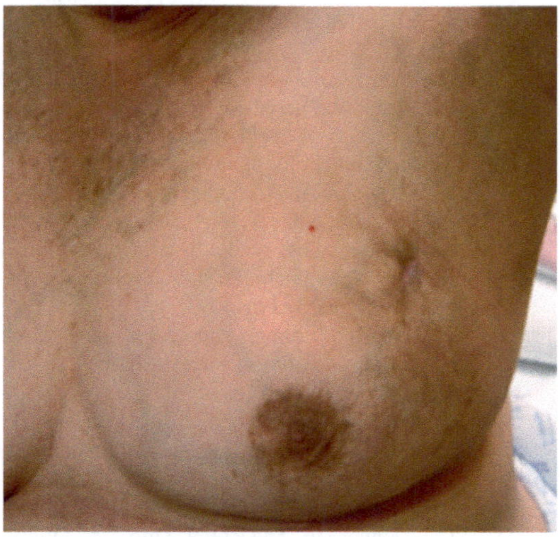

Fig. 1.13 Six months after FAC. Complete clinical response

a recent randomized clinical trial evaluating women with locally advanced breast cancer that included 63 women with IBC evaluated the addition of 1 year of trastuzumab among women with HER2-positive disease; the results favored the group receiving trastuzumab [32].

Despite progress in combined modality treatment with chemotherapy, surgery, and radiation therapy, the long-term outcome for patients with

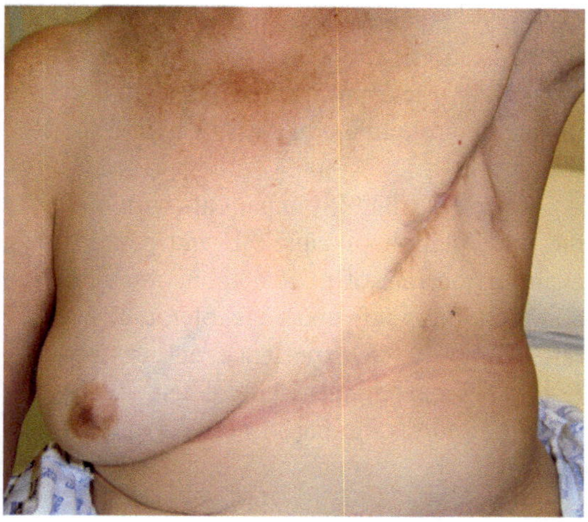

Fig. 1.14 Forty months posttreatment

Inflammatory breast cancer (IBC) remains poor [36]. Therapies that target vascular–lymphatic processes have shown potential in the treatment of IBC, as represented by bevacizumab.

In one study, 21 patients with inflammatory and locally advanced breast cancer [37] were treated with bevacizumab for one cycle (15 mg/kg on day 1) followed by six cycles of bevacizumab with doxorubicin (50 mg/m^2) and docetaxel (75 mg/m^2) every 3 weeks. After locoregional therapy, patients received eight cycles of bevacizumab alone, in addition to hormonal therapy when indicated. During treatment, tumor biopsies and dynamic contrast-enhanced magnetic resonance imaging (DCE-MRI) were performed; this treatment showed a median decrease of 66.7 % in phosphorylated VEGFR2 (Y951) in tumor cells ($p=0.004$), and a median increase of 128.9 % in tumor apoptosis ($p=0.0008$) was observed after bevacizumab alone, and these changes persisted with the addition of chemotherapy. The authors conclude that bevacizumab exerts inhibitory effects on VEGF receptor activation and vascular permeability and induces apoptosis in tumor cells; however, additional studies are required to understand and demonstrate the benefit of this therapy.

Therapies that target cell proliferation pathways are the most promising targeted therapies for IBC. In particular, therapies that target human EGFR 2, such as trastuzumab and lapatinib, have exhibited good performance in the clinical setting, leading to improved outcomes for patients with IBC. Metastatic pathways could play a unique key role in the aggressiveness of the IBC phenotype.

A phase II trial [38] in patients with IBC with the combination of lapatinib and paclitaxel to evaluate the rate of pCR demonstrates that the combination is safe and well-tolerated; the pCR rate was 18.2 % experience at our institute. Eighty percent patients were treated with anthracycline- and taxane-based neoadjuvant chemotherapy; the remaining patients received chemotherapy without anthracyclines; and 45 % of these patients also received preoperative radiotherapy. Overall, cPR was achieved in 15 % of cases. At a median 24-month follow-up, 61 % of patients had disease relapse, with 13 % local recurrence and the remainder, systemic recurrence; the main recurrence site was lung, central nervous system (CNS), and liver, and median disease-free survival (DFS) was 39 %. At the same follow-up time, 27 % of patients had died due to progressive disease. We conducted an analysis of subgroups according to pathologic response, classifying these as complete response and residual disease. We found that the cPR group had a median survival of 76 % compared with the group with residual disease; median survival was 32 % (log-rank, 0.029), and we also carried out an analysis according to immunohistochemistry (IHC) subgroup, finding a median DFS of 25.9, 45, and 45.7 % in triple-negative, HER2-positive, and ER-positive tumors, respectively, without statistical significance (log-rank = 0.141).

In this book, we have attempted to provide you with updated information taken from the review of multiple recently published articles by leaders in this field. We are aware that there are probably hundreds of publications on inflammatory breast cancer, but this information is, in the majority of the cases, fragmented, and additionally, the results are reported together with those for patients with locally advanced breast cancer.

References

1. Cristofanilli M, Buzdar A, Hortobagyi GN. Update on the management of inflammatory breast cancer. Oncologist. 2003;8:141–8.
2. Haagensen C. Diseases of the breast, 3rd ed. Philadelphia: WB Saunders, 1986:663.
3. Hansen KW, Anderson WF, Devesa SS, et al. Trends in inflammatory breast carcinoma incidence and survival: the surveillance, epidemiology and end results program at the National Cancer Institute. J Natl Cancer Inst. 2005;97:966–75.
4. SEER cancer statistics were updated on 10 Nov 2011. NCI. USA.
5. Boussen H, Bouzaiene H, Ben Hassouna J, et al. Inflammatory breast cancer in Tunisia: epidemiological and clinical trends. Cancer. 2010;116:2730–5.
6. American Joint Committee on Cancer (AJCC) 7th Edition of Cancer Staging Manual, October 14, 2009.
7. Dawood S, Merajver SD, Viens P, et al. International expert panel on inflammatory breast cancer: consensus statement for standardized diagnosis and treatment. Ann Oncol. 2010. doi:10.1093/annonc/mdq345.
8. Bonnier P, Charpin C, Lejeune C, et al. Inflammatory carcinomas of the breast: a clinical, pathological or a clinical and pathological definition? Int J Cancer. 1995;62:382.
9. Cristofanilli M, Buzdar AU, et al. The evaluation of p53, HER2/neu, and serial MDR protein expression as possible markers of chemoresistance and their use as prognostic markers in inflammatory breast cancer. (Abstract). Proc Am Soc Clin Oncol. 1998;17:553a.
10. Aziz SA, Pervez S, Khan S, et al. Case control study of prognostic markers and disease outcome in inflammatory carcinoma breast: unique clinical experience. Breast J. 2001;7:398–404.
11. Soussi T. The *p53* tumor suppressor gene: from molecular biology to clinical investigation. Ann N Y Acad Sci. 2000;910:121–37.
12. Moll UM, LaQuaglia M, Benard J, et al. Wild type p53 protein undergoes cytoplasmic sequestration in undifferentiated neuroblastomas but not in differentiated tumors. Proc Natl Acad Sci USA. 1995;92:4407–11.
13. Mayo LD, Donner DB. The PTEN, Mdm2, p53 tumor suppressor-oncoprotein network. Trends Biochem Sci. 2002;27:462–7.
14. Ann WG, Chuman Y, Fojo T, et al. Inhibitors of transcription proteasome inhibitors and DNA-damaging drugs differentially affect feedback of *p53* degradation. Exp Cell Res. 1998;244:54–60.
15. Berx G, Van Roy F. The E-cadherin/catenin complex: an important gatekeeper in breast cancer tumorigenesis and malignant progression. Breast Cancer Res. 2001;3:289–93.
16. Kleer CG, van Golen KL, Braun T, et al. Persistent E-cadherin expression in inflammatory breast cancer. Mod Pathol. 2001;14:458–64.

17. Tomlinson JS, Alpaugh ML, Barsky SH. An intact overexpressed E-cadherin/alpha, beta-catenin axis characterizes the lymphovascular emboli of inflammatory breast carcinoma. Cancer Res. 2001;61:5231–41.
18. Muller A, Homey B, Soto H, et al. Involvement of chemokine receptors in breast cancer metastases. Nature. 2001;410:50–6.
19. Kijowski J, Baj-Kryzworzeka M, Majka M, et al. The SDF-1-CXCR4 axis stimulates VEGF secretion and activates integrins but does not effect proliferation and survival in lymphohematopoietic cells. Stem Cells. 2001;19:453–66.
20. Bachelder R, Wendt M, Mercurio A. Vascular endothelial growth factor promotes breast carcinoma invasion in an autocrine manner by regulating the chemokine receptor CXCR4. Cancer Res. 2002;62:7203–6.
21. Cabioglu N, Summy J, Miller C, et al. CXCL-12/stromal cell-derived factor-1 alpha transactivates HER2-*neu* in breast cancer cells by a novel pathway involving Src kinase activation. Cancer Res. 2005;65:6493–7.
22. Sallusto F, Lenig D, Forster R, et al. Two subsets of memory T lymphocytes with distinct homing potentials and effector functions. Nature. 1999;401:708–12.
23. Cabioglu N, Gong Y, Islam R, et al. Expression of growth factor and chemokine receptors: new insights in the biology of inflammatory breast cancer. Ann Oncol. 2007;18:1021–9.
24. Parton M, Dowsett M, Ashley S, et al. High incidence of HER-2 positivity in inflammatory breast cancer. Breast. 2004;13:97–103.
25. Sawaki M, Ito Y, Akiyama F, et al. High prevalence of HER-2/*neu* and *p53* overexpression in inflammatory breast cancer. Breast Cancer. 2006;13:172–8.
26. Troester MA, Lee MH, Carter M, et al. Activation of host wound responses in breast cancer microenvironment. Clin Cancer Res. 2009;15:7020–8.
27. Van Laere S, Beissbarth T, Van der Auwera I, et al. Relapse-free survival in breast cancer patients is associated with a gene expression signature characteristic for inflammatory breast cancer. Clin Cancer Res. 2008;14:7452–60.
28. Van Laere S, Van der Auwera I, Van den Eynden GG, et al. Distinct molecular signature of inflammatory breast cancer by cDNA microarray analysis. Breast Cancer Res Treat. 2005;3:237–46.
29. Ueno NT, Buzdar AU, Singletary SE, et al. Combined-modality treatment of inflammatory breast carcinoma: twenty years of experience at M.D. Anderson Cancer Center. Cancer Chemother Pharmacol. 1997;40:321–9.
30. Cristofanilli M, González-Angulo AM, Buzdar AU, et al. Paclitaxel improves the prognosis in estrogen receptor negative inflammatory breast cancer: the M.D. Anderson Cancer Center experience. Clin Breast Cancer. 2004;4:415–9.
31. Veyret C, Levy C, Chollet P, et al. Inflammatory breast cancer outcome with epirubicin-based induction and maintenance chemotherapy: ten-year results from the French Adjuvant Study Group GETIS 02 trial. Cancer. 2006;107:2535–44.
32. Cheng YC, Rondon G, Yang Y, et al. The use of high-dose cyclophosphamide, carmustine, and thiotepa plus autologous hematopoietic stem cell transplantation as consolidation therapy for high-risk primary breast cancer after primary surgery or neoadjuvant chemotherapy. Biol Blood Marrow Transplant. 2004;10:794–804.
33. Gianni L, Eiermann W, Semiglazov V, et al. Neoadjuvant chemotherapy with trastuzumab followed by adjuvant trastuzumab versus neoadjuvant chemotherapy alone, in patients with HER2-positive locally advanced breast cancer (the NOAH trial): a randomised controlled superiority trial with a parallel HER2-negative cohort. Lancet. 2010;375(9712):377–84.
34. Bristol IJ, Woodward WA, Strom EA, et al. Locoregional treatment outcomes after multimodality management of inflammatory breast cancer. Int J Radiat Oncol Biol Phys. 2008;72:474–84.
35. Panades M, Olivotto IA, Speers CH. Evolving treatment strategies for inflammatory breast cancer. J Clin Oncol. 2005;23:1941–50.
36. Yamauchi H, Cristofanilli M, Nakamura S, et al. Molecular targets for treatment of inflammatory breast cancer. Nat Rev Clin Oncol. 2009;6:387–94.
37. Wedam SB, Low JA, Yang SX, et al. Antiangiogenic and antitumor effects of bevacizumab in patients with inflammatory and locally advanced breast cancer. J Clin Oncol. 2006;24:769–77.
38. Boussen H, Cristofanilli M, Zaks T, et al. Phase II study to evaluate the efficacy and safety of neoadjuvant lapatinib plus placlitaxel in patients with inflammatory breast cancer. J Clin Oncol. 2010;28:3248–55.

2 Breast Cancer: Epidemiological Panorama and Opportunities for Prevention

Nancy Reynoso-Noveron
and Alejandro Mohar-Betancourt

Introduction

Breast cancer has been described from very ancient times. However, given the changes observed worldwide in demographic and epidemiological patterns over several recent decades, the appearance of cases of nontransmittable diseases – linked with the aging of the population and adherence to unhealthy lifestyles – has produced an epidemic pattern in their incidence, including breast cancer.

Breast cancer is at present the most frequently found malignant tumor among women throughout the world. It has also been described as the first cause of death for this population group, making it one of the diseases with the greatest social and economic impact in our times. It represents a serious health problem and one of the most complex challenges of health systems.

The knowledge generated surrounding this problem has been fundamental for offering patients with breast cancer the best care possible. Notwithstanding this, differences in survival among different regions of the world continue to be substantial. Thus, a narration of the epidemiology of the disease addressed to the health personnel charged with the diagnosis, management, and control of the disease will motivate us all to continue working in the search for novel opportunities for its prevention and early detection, a strategy also useful in the control of diseases as poignant as breast cancer.

The purpose of this chapter, in addition to showing the tendencies in the appearance of cases in the world and specifically in Mexico, is to describe the conditions that have been associated with the appearance of the disease, the transcendence of an early diagnosis, and the characteristics related with the survival of those afflicted with the disease. In addition, the importance of screening programs and the difficulties in carrying these out in developing countries such as Mexico will be described. Finally, we present a recapitulation of present and future challenges in health systems with the purpose of reducing the morbimortality of this frequently occurring neoplasm.

N. Reynoso-Noveron, M.D., Ph.D.
Unidad de Investigación Biomédica en Cáncer,
Instituto Nacional de Cancerología (INCan),
Universidad Nacional Autónoma de México (UNAM),
Mexico City, DF, Mexico

A. Mohar-Betancourt, M.D., Ph.D. (✉)
Department of General Direction,
Instituto Nacional de Cancerología,
San Fernando Number 22, Tlalpan,
Mexico City, DF 14080, Mexico
e-mail: amohar@incan.edu.mx

J.G. de la Garza-Salazar et al. (eds.), *Inflammatory Breast Cancer*,
DOI 10.1007/978-0-85729-991-8_2, © Springer-Verlag London 2013

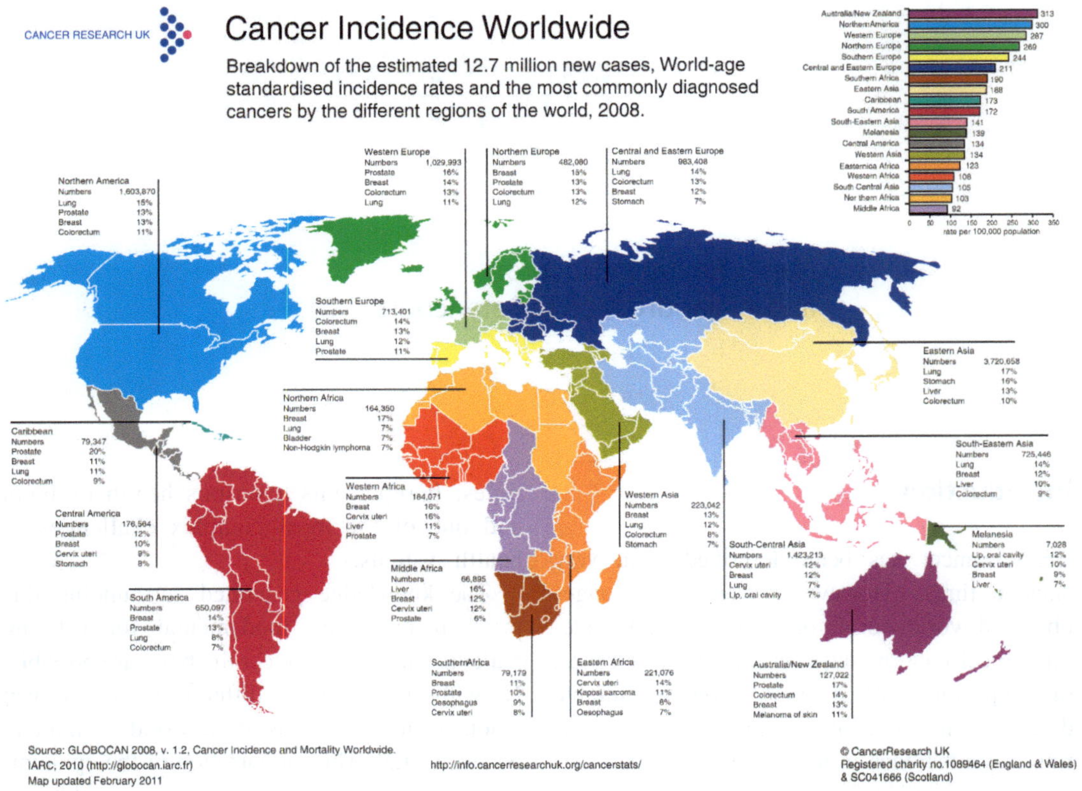

Fig. 2.1 Cancer incidence worldwide, International Agency for Research on Cancer (*IARC*), Cancer Research UK, http://info.cancerresearchuk.org/cancerstats/world/the-global-picture/, April 2012

World Panorama

According to the World Cancer Report 2000, the incidence of cancer at any localization would increase by 50 % by the year 2020, in which there would be 15 million new cases. In 2000, malignant tumors were the cause of 12 % of nearly 56 million deaths that were produced throughout the world; in many countries, more than one-quarter of these deaths were attributable to cancer. In that same year, 5.3 million males and 4.7 million females presented malignant tumors. Likewise, there were 6.2 million cancer-related deaths.

This same report in 2008 informed 12.4 million new cases of cancer, with 7.6 million deaths worldwide. More than one-half of the cases and 60 % of deaths took place in developing countries, with the greatest incidence reported in North America, Australia, and in Northern and Western Europe (Fig. 2.1). The highest rates were observed for breast cancer and prostate cancer, followed by cancer of the lung, stomach, colon and rectum, liver, and uterine cervix, being these the most frequent cancers in the world [1].

Breast cancer is the most frequent malignant tumor in women worldwide, with only 15–30 % of cases corresponding to carcinomas in situ and the remainder to infiltrating carcinomas. In addition, 90 % of carcinomas develop in the ductal epithelium, and 10 % affect the lobular tissue of the breast [2]. In 2008, it was estimated that 1.38 million new cases were diagnosed, which corresponded to 23 % of all causes of cancer identified in females and 10.9 % of all cancers at the general level, that is, also considering the masculine population.

The incidence rate of breast cancer is high in developed countries, where more than one-half of cases are concentrated, nearly 36,000 in Europe (27.3 % of the cancers of women in this region) and 230,000 in North America (31.3 %). Only in Japan does breast cancer occupy third place after

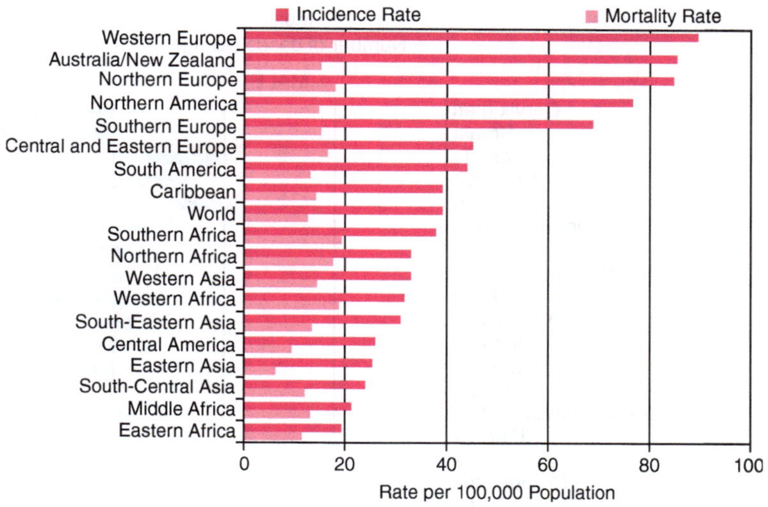

Fig. 2.2 Incidence rate and standardized regional mortality by age of breast cancer, International Agency for Research on Cancer (*IARC*), 2008 (Ferlay et al. [8])

colorectal cancer and cancer of the stomach. The highest age-standardized incidence rate is found in North America, with an incidence of 99.4/100,000 inhabitants, together with some other countries in South America such as Brazil and Argentina, in addition to those of Northwestern Europe and Australia. A moderate incidence has been observed in Eastern Europe, South America, Southern Africa, and Western Asia, but even so, breast cancer in these regions continues to be the most common cancer found among women, and low rates have been described for the populations of Asia and Africa, although recently an increase has been reported in the number of cases in these regions [3, 4].

The World Health Organization (WHO) has described significant changes in the profile of this epidemic; after having arisen in the most developed regions of the planet, it is now affecting in a growing manner women in countries with lesser resources [5]. From the year 2000, breast cancer became the most frequent tumor among women of low-income countries, places where cancer of the uterine cervix had been the leader during the past two decades.

With respect to mortality, breast cancer has been situated in the fifth place as cause of death among all neoplastic diseases, but in the first place in feminine population worldwide (269,000 deaths, 12.7 % of the total) in developing as well as in developed countries. Survival in patients with breast cancer has increased little by little in developed countries, with reports of up to 89 % for the USA [6], while developing countries continue to show survival rates of <50 % [7] (Fig. 2.2).

From 1990, differences in the incidence and mortality of this disease among regions in the entire world were glimpsed, suggesting an important role for environmental factors in the susceptibility for developing cancer for certain populations. The latter has been expressed through some studies conducted in migrant population in which the increase was clearly shown of the risk for having cancer in populations originating in countries with low incidences, such as Italy or Poland, when these have migrated at early ages to countries with a high disease rate, such as Australia [9, 10]. Similarly, on comparing risks in the children of migrants, an increase has been shown in the risk of presenting the disease in the first, second, and third generations [11].

Given the regional differences, some authors describe reproductive factors such as low parity, late age at first pregnancy, obesity, and nutrition as factors that are crucial for the appearance of breast cancer [12]. It has been established that contrasts in mortality rates among the different regions are much less marked than those described regarding incidence rates, which could be the effect of efficient early detection programs in fully developed countries.

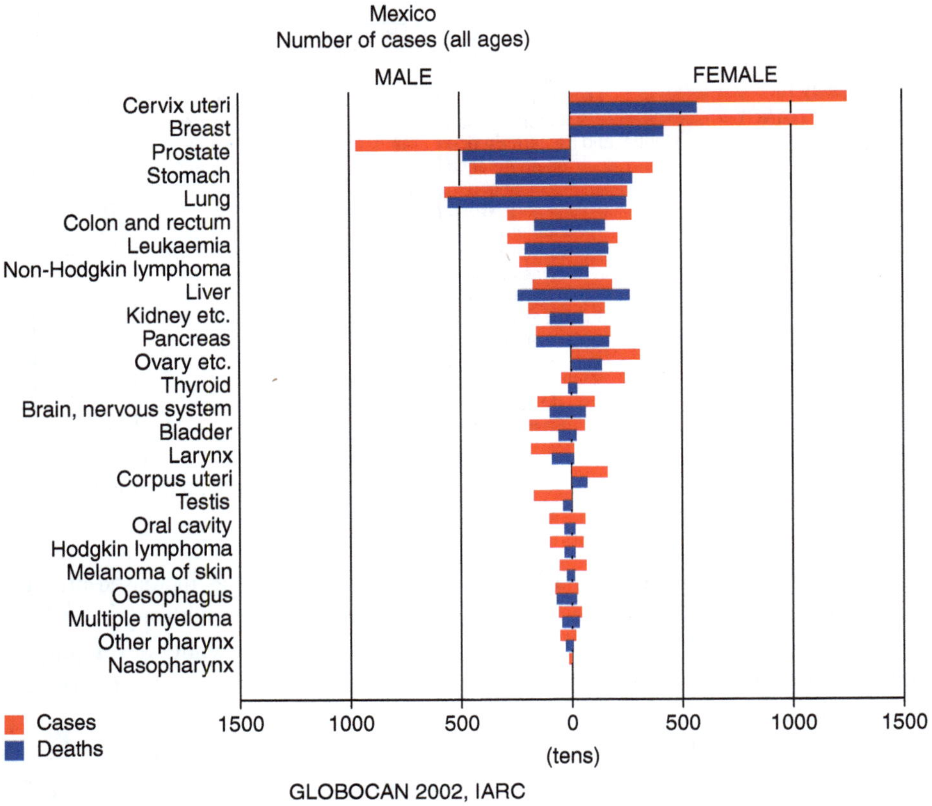

Fig. 2.3 Number of cases and deaths due to cancer in Mexico according to gender, International Agency for Research on Cancer (*IARC*), 2002 (Ferlay et al. [8])

National Panorama

In Mexico, the main neoplastic diseases that affect the masculine population are cancer of the prostate, lung, stomach, leukemias, and colorectal cancer. In women, cancer of the breast, uterine cervix, stomach, liver, and colorectal cancer cause the greatest burden that the country sustains due to this group of diseases [13] (Fig. 2.3).

According to the International Agency for Research on Cancer (IARC), Mexico occupies 101st place in incidence and 135th place in breast cancer-associated deaths of the 172 countries with available epidemiological information. Breast cancer in Mexico has occupied first place in deaths since 2006 due to malignant neoplasms in women, exceeding cervical cancer, which historically occupied first place (Fig. 2.4). The age-adjusted mortality rate reported in Mexico has been important: from 5.9/100,000 in 1980 to nearly nine million in the mid-1990s. For 2007, a rate was notified of 16.5 deaths/100,000 women aged 25 years and over. In 2008, the incidence of breast cancer in Mexico was reported as 7.57 cases/100,000 women 15 years of age and over. In Mexico, this disease is more important in the northern and central states with lower rates in southern states that although these are entities with low socioeconomic levels, they also have breast cancer among the main causes of mortality [14].

Similarly to the rest of the world, the number of cases and the mortality rate also rise with age in Mexico. However, the appearance has been reported of new cases at early ages, which contrasts with those registered in the USA and Europe, where the greatest incidence presents in postmenopausal women aged 50 years or more [15].

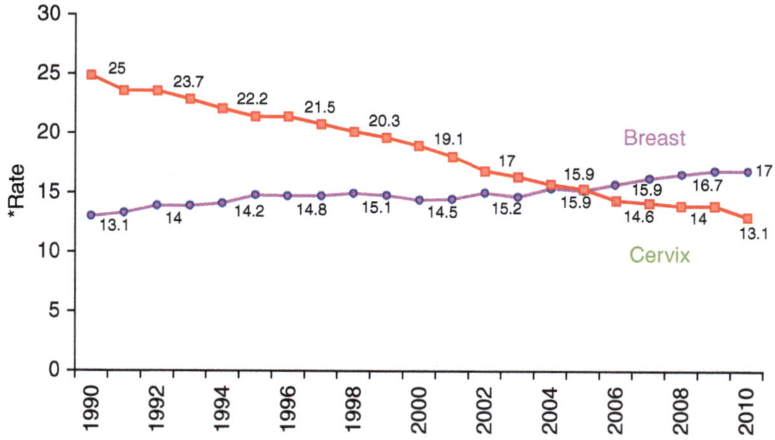

*Rate per 100,000 women aged 25 years and over
**Preliminary data Directorate General of Health Information (DGIS, Salud México) 2010

Fig. 2.4 National cancer of the uterine cervix- and breast-cancer-related trends in mortality rates, 1990–2010**. (Figure modified from National Institute of Statistics and Geography (*INEGI*)/ Ministry of Health (*SSA*))

Risk Factors

While the causes and natural history of the disease have not been completely defined, it is recognized that age is the principal risk factor for the development of neoplastic processes. Breast cancer is no exception, with the risk for women >30 years of age ten times greater than that of those aged <20 years, with a proportional increase that reaches >90 times in women of >60 years of age [16]. At the same time, the greatest frequency of this disease has been described among women of high socioeconomic status, those who reside in urban zones, and among those who had never been married.

Other data from epidemiological researches describe the association of some genetic, biological, and environmental factors as cofactors for development of the disease. The prevalence and distribution of risk factors in diverse countries of Latin America and the Caribbean are depicted in Fig. 2.5 and comprise the following:

- Genetic factors. It is known that women who have a direct relative (mother, sister, or daughter) in whom breast cancer has been diagnosed have double the risk of developing the disease. Approximately 10 % of women with breast cancer report having a relative with the same disease, and among these, some present *BRCA1* and *BRCA2* mutations. The risk of developing cancer in the presence of these alterations is 80 %; although it has been described that the absolute risk can vary according to the country of residence [17], the hereditary characteristic of this disease generally accompanies the diagnosis of this at early ages between 30 and 50 years and multiple cases of early-onset breast or ovarian cancer in the family [18, 19].
- Fetal exposure. It has been described that women whose birth weight was >4 kg had a 3.5 times greater risk of developing breast cancer than those who weighed <3 kg at birth; this association has been described in many women who present a diagnosis prior to menopause. This is explained as due to the estrogen levels that determine the size of the placenta related with the fetal growth rate; thus, babies with overweight are also exposed to greater amounts of maternal estrogens [20–22].
- Reproductive factors. The time span from menarche to the birth of the first child also results as a vulnerable period for mammary tissue. The mammary gland terminates its development once pregnancy and lactation are over; therefore, an undifferentiated breast is more sensitive to carcinogens than a completely differentiated breast [23]. Additionally, it has been described that the risk for breast cancer diminishes with the number of deliveries; after the first of these, the risk diminishes by 7 % for each child; likewise, lactation

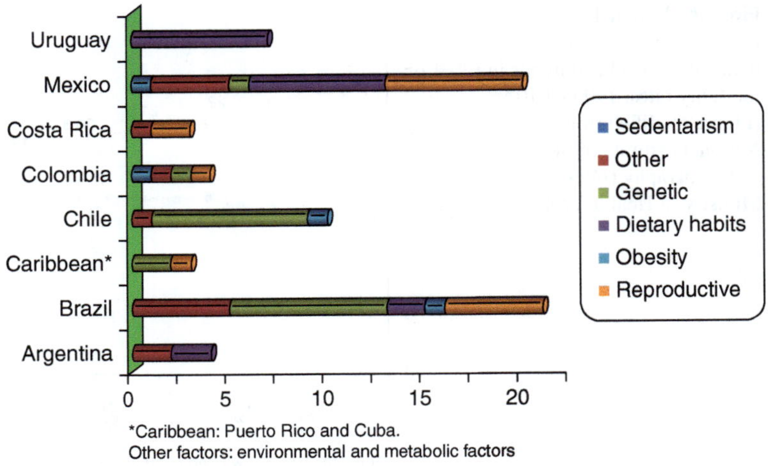

Fig. 2.5 Risk factors in breast cancer in Latin America and the Caribbean (Figure modified from Cancer de mama, Tomatelo a Pecho 2009. Mexican Health Foundation (*FUNSALUD*)/National Public Health Institute (*INSP*))

diminishes by 5 % the risk of developing the disease for each year that the woman breastfeeds. Also, although breast cells proliferate at the middle of the menstrual cycle, these, once pregnancy does not take place, suffer from apoptosis; the number of times that this occurs has also been associated with a higher risk for developing breast cancer. This is one of the reasons that early menarche or very late menopause has also been observed to be related [24].

- External use of hormones. It has been recognized that the use of hormonal contraceptives increases the risk of developing breast cancer by 7 %, this compared with nonexposed women. It has been described that there is no increase in risk in menopausal women who are users of this type of contraceptives, as well as there being no effect on mortality due to breast cancer in these women who use hormonal contraceptives [25]. Evolution of the use of hormones during or after menopause and its relation with the appearance of cancer has given rise to contradictory results. The most recent data confirm that the risk increases depending on hormone type and duration of use; hormones solely based on estrogens do not increase the risk [26, 27].
- Alcohol and obesity. It has also been described that the daily consumption of 24 g of alcohol increases the risk for breast cancer by 21 %, which can be explained as due to the diminution of the hepatic metabolism of the estrogens of the alcohol-drinking woman. On the other hand, it is known that adipose tissue is a source of the formation of estrogens; thus, there is a strong correlation between the amount of adipose tissue and estrogen levels in postmenopausal women. Women with a body mass index (BMI) of 27 or more have a 40 % greater risk of presenting breast cancer [28, 29].
- Physical activity and diet. Several studies have shown a diminution in the risk for cancer when physical activity increases; it has even been described that women engaging in at least 30 min of exercise daily reduce the risk of presenting the disease by 50 % compared with women with a sedentary lifestyle. Greater intake of fruits and vegetables is stipulated as being able to cause a reduction in the risk of presenting the disease; it has been inconsistently described that greater intake of vegetables can prevent breast cancer in young women and that low intake of fats can probably exert a preventive impact in postmenopausal women [30–33].

In this context, it is noteworthy that the demographic and epidemiological transition that the population has undergone has given rise to that some of the factors, described previously, contribute to the increase in the frequency of this disease, mainly those linked with an unhealthy lifestyle—lack of exercise, an unhealthy diet, and an increase in alcohol consumption—all of which are potentially modifiable factors [34]. These findings, added to the delay in the time of the first pregnancy and the increase in life expectancy, explain the increase in the incidence of breast cancer observed during the past decades.

Diagnosis

Although the description of diagnostic techniques and treatment strategies lies outside of the objective of this chapter, we must remember that diagnostic and treatment strategies have changed throughout the history of breast cancer. At the beginning of the 1960s, when the use of the first mammographies had recently begun, a radical mastectomy was the predominant therapy, and this did not change with the patient's clinical stage or characteristics. At present, there is conservative breast surgery, intraoperative radiotherapy, and hormonal and biological therapy.

Diagnostic techniques have been strengthened in the last 40 years, attempting to cover the need for detecting small tumors of millimetric dimensions [35]. The diagnosis of breast cancer depends on whether the lesion is palpable or not. If the lesion is palpable, diagnosis is performed by means of inspection and palpation, mammography, or biopsy. Nonpalpable lesions present a greater diagnostic challenge; under this circumstance, a suspicious lesion is localized through special mammographic techniques or ultrasonography, and biopsies are carried out by orientation of imaging techniques. The breast represents a true challenge in obtaining its x-ray image; a screening mammography seeks out nonpalpable lesions (i.e., <0.3 cm), microcalcifications, asymmetries in mammary density, and/or distortion of the structure of the gland. The American College of Radiology (ACR) created a classification system denominated BI-RADS (Breast Imaging Reporting and Data System), which aids in standardizing and reducing the possible confusion of mammographic images [36]. The mastography permits the visualization of these indicators, but the gravity of the lesion is determined solely by histopathological analysis.

Prognostic Factors

The management of breast cancer requires a multidisciplinary team and a great investment of the health systems that allows covering the very high cost of antineoplastic drugs, which sometimes is not always reflected in an improvement in the survival rates of this specific population group. As mentioned previously, the 5-year global survival of patients with breast cancer exhibits sufficiently heterogeneous data within the different world regions. The most recent data in the USA describes 5-year survival rates of up to 89 %, while in Europe, this ranges from 22.7 % in Italy to 46.5 % reported for Spain [37].

Among factors known to affect patients' survival, we find mainly clinical stage at the moment of diagnosis; survival will be less if at the time of diagnosis, the cancer is found in an advanced stage. Considering all of the races, survival data have been reported of 98 % for localized disease, of 84 % for regional disease, and of 23 % for infiltrating disease. Survival diminishes according to the size of the tumor; in regional disease, 5-year survival comes to be up to 95 % for tumors <2.0 cm, 82 % for tumors from 2.1 to 5.0 cm, and up to 66 % for tumors >5 cm [38].

Another factor that is known to affect survival is the age of the woman at the time of diagnosis. If this occurs prior to 40 years of age, reported survival is of 83 % compared with those whose diagnosis was performed after this age, whose survival is described as 90 %. One proposed explanation is that, in general, tumors diagnosed in young women tend to be more aggressive and as having a lesser response to treatment [39].

There are also reports showing that Afro-American women have a lesser probability of 5-year survival after a diagnosis of breast cancer than Caucasian women, 78 versus 90 %, respectively. This difference can be explained as much by advanced stage as by poor definition of the stage at the time of diagnosis.

Finally, it is also known that the lack of access to primary health-care services is associated with low survival among patients with cancer. Likewise, women from low socioeconomic strata have a lower possibility of 5-year survival than those in high strata [40].

Early Detection

At the worldwide level, stage at diagnosis varies substantially. In the USA, for example, the prevalence of metastatic breast cancer at the time of diagnosis is low, around 3.35 % [41], while in Europe, the proportion of new cases in women diagnosed with advanced disease ranges between 3 and 11 %, although for Germany, the proportion of detection of cases of women in advanced stages is around 15 % [37, 42–47], while in Mexico, around 75 % of cases detected are found in women in advanced disease stages [48]. The low proportion of cases detected at early stages, when the probability of 5-year survival is very much higher if adequate treatment is received, is the cause that most cases have a poor prognosis, and in turn, the medical care required is more complex and highly expensive. As previously explained, contrasts in disease incidence and survival between developing and developed countries can be due to the success in the instrumentation of screening programs for achieving the increase of the detection of sick patients at the beginning of the disease. Thus, providing treatment in timely fashion improves the quality of life of the patients and reduces the expenditure for the care of this disease.

Among timely detection techniques, breast self-examination based on observation and palpation that the woman herself performs on her own breasts is recommended by the American Cancer Society (ACS) to be carried out monthly in all women from the menarche, above all in women >20 years of age. Some studies describe this technique as a useless tool for detecting early lesions. In Mexico, there are diverse publications in this respect in which it is concluded that women are capable of detecting lesions of at least 1 cm and when these are superficial, and even of 0.5 cm once they have received training in this technique [49].

The worldwide impact of breast self-examination shows inconsistent data and apparently does not offer an impact on the diminution of mortality. Other reports refer a better prognosis for patients because lesions are detected in clinical stages I and II [50]. In Mexico, 90 % of cases of breast cancer are detected because the patient herself detects a lump or node, and in the majority of these cases, this comprises an advanced disease stage [48].

The mammography is the most utilized diagnostic tool at the worldwide level in screening programs and in the diagnosis of breast cancer; notwithstanding this, the effectiveness of breast self-examination and clinical examination in the mortality of this disease remains an issue for debate in relation to their usefulness as auxiliary diagnostic tools in developing countries, where carrying out mammographic studies is unfeasible [51, 52]. In Mexico, mammographies have been employed nearly fully with diagnostic purposes; it was in 2003 that Official Mexican Norm 041-SSA2-2002 for the prevention, diagnosis, treatment, and control of breast cancer opened the possibility for use of the mammography for the purpose of screening of the population [53].

There are several studies that have evaluated the effect of screening with mammography in the reduction of mortality rates for this disease, observing a diminution that ranges from 28 to 65 % with a mean of 46 % [54–56]. In 2002, the International Agency for Research of Cancer (IARC) concluded that there is sufficient evidence supplied by clinical assays on the effect of screening on the mortality of women between 50 and 69 years of age with breast cancer. A reduction was notified of 25 % in the mortality of this neoplasm on analysis by protocol and of 35 % in intent-to-treat analysis in all women who had regular mammographies. Some studies cite that the effectiveness of the test was greater in the group of women aged 50–69 years than in that of women aged 40–49 years, with a diminution in

Most Recently Published Results of the Breast Cancer Screening Trial son Breast Cancer Mortality Reduction With invitation to Screening

Study	Age Range	Percentage Mortality Reduction (95%CI)**
HIP	40–64	24(7,38)
Malmö	45–69	19(–8,39)
Two-Country Trial, Sweden	40–74	32(20,41)
Edinburgh	45–64	21(–2,40)
Stockholm	40–64	26(–10,50)
Canada NB SS-1	40–49	–3(–26,27)
Canada NB SS-2	50–59	–2(–33,22)
Gothenburg	39–59*	16(–39,49)
All Trials Combined	39–74	24(18,30)

*There are more recent publications from the Gothenburg trial but they refer only to the under 50 age group

**CI = Confidence interval

Fig. 2.6 Results of recently published assays in which the reduction in mortality by means of screening programs was evaluated. American Cancer Society (*ACS*) 2003 (Figure modified from Smith Robert et al. [62])

the mortality rate of 16–35 and 15–20 %, respectively [51]. The beneficial effect for the group aged between 40 and 49 years remains controversial [52, 57]. The ACS recommends a screening mammogram every year for women 40 years of age and over, and the American Medical Association (AMA) and the National Cancer Institute (NCI) recommend a screening mammography once every 1 or 2 years for women between the ages of 40 and 49 years and an annual mammography from the age of 50 years. The Canadian Cancer Society (CCS) recommends that women aged between 50 and 59 years have a mammography and a clinical breast examination once every 2 years [58].

In Sweden, the recommendation for women between 50 and 69 years is for submittal to screening mammographies without indicating the frequency. Recently, the US Preventive Services Task Force (USPSTF) recommended that the decision for carrying out mammography in women aged from 40 to 49 years should be approached together with the physician, taking into account the risk factors and the patient's preference [59, 60], showing the need for studies that support the decision of the best age at which, and the specific criteria for which, women should be submitted to a screening mammography because, on the other hand, the risk of radio inducing a cancer in women with a genetic predisposition has also been recognized in other scientific researches [61] (Fig. 2.6).

Therefore, although screening has been proposed as the main strategy for improving the survival of patients with breast cancer, the impact of this type of program exerted on developing countries has been low due perhaps to limited coverage of women at high risk [63]. It may also be due to the deficient quality in the medical care process and to the lack of homologation of diagnostic criteria due to lack of quality control and ongoing training systems of its personnel, but also to multifactorial obstacles—social, cultural, geographic, economic, behavioral, familial, and organizational—which have already been described, such as imprecise knowledge of breast cancer and detection methods, the inexistence of data on knowledge on and attitudes toward breast cancer, above all in minority groups, scarce awareness concerning early detection, lack of medical insurance covering mammographic detection, and lack of instruction on early detection and related programs. All of these are factors impede breast cancer from being identified and diagnosed at the earliest stages, when cancer treatment may be effectively and efficiently administered [64, 65].

Prevention

Despite that the management of breast cancer has been surprising in recent years and that strategies have been proposed for early detection of the disease in order to improve the prognosis of patients already suffering from the disease, strong contrasts continue today in the world with respect to success in control of the disease. This is due to the deficiencies in medical coverage and sociocultural barriers that limit timely detection and treatment in developing countries.

Notwithstanding the latter, speaking out on primary prevention of breast cancer is inexistent and even controversial. While we are not completely sure at present of the manner by which and magnitude at which we can come to prevent the development of malignant lesions in mammary tissue, we do know the potentially modifiable risk factors that are associated with its appearance. Thus, in addition to fortifying timely detection and medical care for patients who already have the disease, we should promote regular physical activity, maintenance of the ideal weight, low alcohol intake, maternal lactation, and rational use of hormone replacement in postmenopausal patients. In addition to this, there are studies, although in debate, that suggest the possibility of applying chemoprevention or even the performance of preventive mastectomy or oophorectomy in women at high risk of having breast cancer [66–72].

Conclusions

The data presented here ratify the magnitude that breast cancer represents as a worldwide epidemic as well as the importance of prevention and offering optimal control for women with this disease.

The control of this disease throughout the world and principally in developing countries is not an easy task. One measurement of control is the intervention of potentially modifiable factors, as well as the registry and epidemiological analysis of the disease, with the purpose of determining risk groups whose members could be submitted to timely screening programs. It is only in this way that we will be able to optimize the limited resources allotted for the control of cancer in Mexico.

According to published in 2008 by Levine P and Veneroso C, the epidemiology of inflammatory breast cancer (IBC) has been of great interest to a number of investigators, but epidemiological research has been hampered by the lack of an agreed upon case definition and the relatively small number of patients available to any single investigator or institution. Several features of IBC have become apparent through population-based studies, which, although varying somewhat in case definition, generally agree on some key features of the disease. These include the incidence of the disease, apparently less than 3 % of breast cancer cases in the USA, the younger age of onset compared to noninflammatory breast cancer, the much higher incidence in Black women compared to White, the generally poor outcome of this disease compared to noninflammatory breast cancer, and the continued increase in reported incidence, particularly as compared with noninflammatory breast cancer in general and locally advanced breast cancer (LABC) in particular. There is an apparent striking geographic pattern, with a higher percentage of cases reported from North Africa, best documented in Tunisia. The risk factors for developing IBC are suggested by smaller studies with concordant conclusions, and some appear to be different than the risk factors for developing breast cancer in general. For example, obesity appears to be a risk factor for premenopausal IBC but is not for premenopausal noninflammatory breast cancer. In addition, there is evidence that a young age at first birth predisposes to IBC but is protective against developing noninflammatory breast cancer. In some malignancies, the use of molecular markers is helpful in defining subgroups that could assist in improving case definition as well as predicting prognosis. The increasing combination of improved epidemiologic and laboratory methods will hopefully accelerate our understanding of this challenging disease [73].

Of course, investment in health coverage, in health promotion, and in the education of medical personnel are basic tasks in health systems to achieve the reduction of the risk for breast cancer and to attain the reduction of the mortality of this so often encountered disease in our environment.

References

1. World Health Organization WHO. International Agency for Research of Cancer. World cancer report. Lyon: IARC Press; 2008. p. 260.
2. Cotran RS, Robbins SL, Kumar V. Patología estructural y funcional. 6th ed. Madrid: McGraw-Hill; 1999.
3. Parkin DM, Whelan SL, Ferlay J, Storm H. Cancer incidence in five continents, vols. 1–8. IARC Cancer Base no. 6. Lyon: IARC Press. Available at: (http://www-dep.iarc.fr). Accessed 25 Nov 2009.
4. Parkin DM, Bray F, Ferlay J, Pisani P. Global cancer statistics, 2002. CA Cancer J Clin. 2005;55:74–108.
5. Organización Mundial de la Salud. Cáncer 2008. Available at: (http://www.who.int/mediacentre/factsheets/fs297/es/index.html). Accessed 25 Oct 2009.
6. Ries LAG, Eisner MP, Kosary CL, et al., editors. SEER cancer statistics review. Bethesda: National Cancer Institute; 2004. p. 1975–2001. Available at: (http://seer.cancer.gov/csr/1975_2001). Accessed 11 Apr 2005.
7. Robles SC, Galanis E. Breast cancer in Latin America and the Caribbean. Rev Panam Salud Publica/Pan Am J Public Health. 2002;11(3):178–84.
8. Ferlay J, Shin HR, Bray F, Forman D, Mathers C and Parkin DM. GLOBOCAN 2008 v1.2, Cancer incidence and mortality worldwide: IARC Cancer Base no. 10 [Internet]. Lyon, France: International Agency for Research on Cancer; 2010. Available from: (http://globocan.iarc.fr). Accessed on 9th December 2011.
9. Geddes M, Parkin DM, Khlat M, Balzi D, Buiatti E, editors. Cancer in Italian migrant populations. Scientific publication no. 123. Lyon: IARC Press; 1993.
10. Tyczynski J, Tarkowski W, Parkin DM, Zatonski W. Cancer mortality among Polish migrants to Australia. Eur J Cancer. 1994;30A:478–84.
11. Ziegler RG, Hoover RN, Pike MC, et al. Migration patterns and breast cancer risk in Asian-American women. J Natl Cancer Inst. 1993;85:1819–27.
12. Kelsey JL, Bernstein L. Epidemiology and prevention of breast cancer. Annu Rev Public Health. 1996;17:47–67.
13. International Agency for Research on Cancer. GLOBOCAN 2002. Available at: (http://www-dep.iarc.fr). Accessed 18 Oct 2008.
14. González-Pier E, Gutiérrez-Delgado C, Stevens G, Barraza-Lloréns M, Porras-Condey R, Carvalho N, et al. Definición de prioridades para las intervenciones de salud en el Sistema de Protección Social en Salud de México. Salud Publica Mex. 2007;49(Supl 1):S37–52.
15. Rodríguez-Cuevas S, Macías CG, Franceschi D, Labastida S. Breast carcinoma presents a decade earlier in Mexican women than in women in the United States or European countries. Cancer. 2001;91:863–8.
16. Forbes JF. The incidence of breast cancer: the global burden, public health considerations. Semin Oncol. 1997;24(1, Suppl 1):S1–20, S1–S35.
17. Collaborative Group on Hormonal Factors in Breast Cancer. Familial breast cancer: collaborative reanalysis of individual data from 52 epidemiological studies including 58,209 women with breast cancer and 101,986 women without the disease. Lancet. 2001; 358:1389–99.
18. Antoniou A, Pharoah PDP, Narod S, Risch HA, Eyfjord JE, Hopper JL, et al. Average risks of breast and ovarian cancer associated with *BRCA1* or *BRCA2* mutations detected in case series unselected for family history: a combined analysis of 22 studies. Am J Hum Genet. 2003;72:1117–30.
19. Narod SA, Foulkes WD. *BRCA1* and *BRCA2*: 1994 and beyond. Nat Rev Cancer. 2004;4:665–76.
20. Trichopoulos D. Is breast cancer initiated in utero? Epidemiology. 1990;1:95–6.
21. Ahlgren M, Sorensen T, Wohlfahrt J, Haflidadottir A, Holst C, Melbye M. Birth weight and risk of breast cancer in a cohort of 106,504 women. Int J Cancer. 2003;107:997–1000.
22. McCormack VA, Silva IDS, Stavola BLD, Mohsen R, León DA, Lithell HO. Fetal growth and subsequent risk of breast cancer: results from long term follow up of Swedish cohort. BMJ. 2003;326:248–53.
23. Vatten LJ, Maehle BO, Nilsen TLL, Tretli S, Hsieh C, Trichopoulos D, Stuver SO. Birth weight as a predictor of breast cancer: a case control study in Norway. Br J Cancer. 2002;86:89–91.
24. Collaborative Group on Hormonal Factors in Breast Cancer. Breast cancer and breastfeeding. Collaborative reanalysis of individual data from 47 epidemiological

studies in 30 countries, including 50 302 women with breast cancer and 96 973 women without the disease. Lancet. 2002;360:187–95.
25. Collaborative Group on Hormonal Factors in Breast Cancer. Breast cancer and hormonal contraceptives. Collaborative reanalysis of individual data on 53 297 women with breast cancer and 100 239 women without breast cancer from 54 epidemiological studies. Collaborative Group on Hormonal Factors in Breast cancer. Lancet. 1996;347:1713–27.
26. Rossouw JE, Anderson GL, Prentice RL, et al. Risks and benefits of estrogen plus progestin in healthy postmenopausal women. Principal results from the Women's Health Initiative randomized controlled trial. JAMA. 2002;288:321–33.
27. Women's Health Initiative Steering Committee. Effects of conjugated equine estrogen in postmenopausal women with hysterectomy. The Women's Health Initiative randomized controlled trial. JAMA. 2004;291:1701–12.
28. Collaborative Group on Hormonal Factors in Breast Cancer. Alcohol, tobacco and breast cancer- collaborative reanalysis of individual data from 53 epidemiological studies, including 58,515 women with breast cancer and 95,067 women without the disease. Br J Cancer. 2002;87:1234–345.
29. Trentham-Dietz A, Newcomb PA, Storer BE, et al. Body size and risk of breast cancer. Am J Epidemiol. 1997;145:1011–9.
30. Thune I, Brenn T, Lund E, Gaard M. Physical activity and the risk of breast cancer. N Engl J Med. 1997; 336:1269–75.
31. Freudenheim JL, Marshall JR, Vena JE, et al. Premenopausal breast cancer risk and intake of vegetables, fruits, and related nutrients. J Natl Cancer Inst. 1996;88:340–8.
32. Furberg AS, Veierod MB, Wilsgaard T, Bernstein L, Thune I. Serum high-density lipoprotein cholesterol, metabolic profile, and breast cancer risk. J Natl Cancer Inst. 2004;96:1152–560.
33. Key TJ, Allen NE, Spencer EA, Travis RC. Nutrition and breast cancer. Breast. 2003;12:412–6.
34. Henderson BE, Bernstein L. The international variation in breast cancer rates: an epidemiological assessment. Breast Cancer Res Treat. 1991;18 Suppl 1:S11–7.
35. Commission of the European Communities. European guidelines for quality assurance in mammography screening, Europe against cancer programme. 3rd ed. Luxembourg: Office for Official Publications of the European Communities; 2001.
36. D'Orsi CJ, et al. Breast imaging reporting and data system (BI-RADS). 4th ed. Reston: ACR; 2003.
37. Sant M, Allemani C, Capocaccia R, et al. Stage at diagnosis is a key explanation of differences in breast cancer survival across Europe. Int J Cancer. 2003; 106(3):416–22.
38. Horner MJ, Ries LAG, Krapcho M, et al., editors. SEER cancer statistics review, 1975–2006. Bethesda: National Cancer Institute; 2009. Available at: http://seer.cancer.gov/csr/1975_2006/, based on November 2008 SEER data submission posted on the SEER web site. Accessed Dec 2011.
39. Anders CK, Hsu DS, Broadwater G, et al. Young age at diagnosis correlates with worse prognosis and defines a subset of breast cancers with shared patterns of gene expression. J Clin Oncol. 2008;26(20):3324–30.
40. Smedley B, Stith A, Nelson A, editors. Unequal treatment: confronting racial and ethnic disparities in health care, Committee on understanding and eliminating racial and ethnic disparities in health care. Washington, D.C.: Institute of Medicine/National Academy Press; 2002.
41. Commission on Cancer – National Cancer Database. Benchmark reports, V 8.0 – 20 Aug, 2007 – STAGE of breast cancer diagnosed in 2004. Commission on Cancer – National Cancer Database (NCDB); 2007.
42. El Saghir NS, Seoud M, Khalil MK, et al. Effects of young age at presentation on survival in breast cancer (Abstract). BMC Cancer. 2006;6:194.
43. Puglisi F, Follador A, Minisini AM, et al. Baseline staging tests after a new diagnosis of breast cancer: further evidence of their limited indications. Ann Oncol. 2005;16(2):263–6.
44. Remak E, Brazil L. Cost of managing women presenting with stage IV breast cancer in the United Kingdom. Br J Cancer. 2004;91(1):77–83.
45. Schneider C, Fehr MK, Steiner RA, Hagen D, Haller U, Fink D. Frequency and distribution pattern of distant metastases in breast cancer patients at the time of primary presentation. Arch Gynecol Obstet. 2003;269(1):9–12.
46. Traina A, Cusimano R, Liquori M, et al. Breast cancer incidence in the city and province of Palermo in 1999–2002: a breast cancer registry report. Ann N Y Acad Sci. 2004;1028:473–80.
47. Efficace F, Biganzoli L, Piccart M, et al. Baseline health-related quality-of-life data as prognostic factors in a phase III multicentre study of women with metastatic breast cancer. Eur J Cancer. 2004;40(7):1021–30.
48. Secretaría de Salud. Subsecretaría de Prevención y Promoción de la Salud. Programa de Acción Específico 2007–2012: Cáncer de mama.
49. Ortega-Altamirano D, López-Cervantes M. Estrategias de la enseñanza de auto examen del Seno en mujeres en edad reproductiva. Salud Publica Mex. 2000;42: 17–25.
50. Millar AB. What is the role of early detection and screening in cancer control? J Public Health Policy. 1993;14(4):403–11.
51. Advisory Committee on Breast Cancer Screening. Screening for breast cancer in England: past and future. NHSBSP publication no. 61. Perth: Typeset by Prepress Projects Ltd. 2006. Available at: (www.prepress-projects.co.uk). Accessed Oct 2008.
52. Tabar L, Yen MF, Vitak B, Chen HHT, Smith RA, Duffy SW. Mammography service screening and mortality in breast cancer patients: 20-year follow-up before and after introduction and screening. Lancet. 2003;361:1405–10.

53. NOM-041-SSA2-2002, Para la prevención, diagnóstico, tratamiento, control y vigilancia epidemiológica del cancer de mama. Diario Oficial, 17 Sept 2003.
54. Humphrey LL, Helfand M, Chan BK, Woolf SH. Breast cancer screening: a summary of the evidence for the U.S. Preventive Services Task Force. Ann Intern Med. 2002;137(5 Part 1):347–60.
55. Fletcher SW, Elmore JG. Clinical practice. Mammographic screening for breast cancer. N Engl J Med. 2003;348(17):1672–80.
56. Pisano ED, Gatsonis C, Hendrick E, Yaffe M, Baum JK, Acharyya S, et al. Diagnostic performance of digital versus film mammography for breast-cancer screening. N Engl J Med. 2005;353(17):1773–83 [Epub 2005 Sep 16].
57. Olsen O, Gozsche PC. Cochrane review on screening for breast cancer with mammography. Lancet. 2001; 358:1340–2.
58. Canadian Cancer Society/National Cancer Institute of Canada. Canadian cancer statistics 2006. Toronto. 2006. Available at: (http://www.cancer.ca). Accessed Dec 2010.
59. Nass S, Ball J, Committee on Improving Mammography Quality Standards, National Cancer Policy Board, Institute of Medicine and National Research Council of the National Academies, editors. Improving breast imaging quality standards. Washington, D.C.: The National Academies Press; 2005.
60. Preventive Services Task Force. Screening for breast cancer. U.S. Preventive Services Task Force recommendation statement. Ann Intern Med. 2009; 151:716–26.
61. Andrieu N, et al. Effect of chest X-rays on the risk of breast cancer among *BRCA1/2* mutation carriers in the international *BRCA1/2* Carrier Cohort Study: a report from the EMBRACE, GENESPO, GEO-HEBON, and IBCCS Collaborator's Group. J Clin Oncol. 2006;24:3361–6.
62. Smith Robert A, et al. American cancer society guidelines for breast cancer screening: update 2003. CA Cancer J Clin. 2003;54:141–69.
63. Mishra SI, Bastani R, Crespi CM, Chang LC, Luc PH, Baquet CR. Results of a randomized trial to increase mammogram usage among Samoan women. Cancer Epidemiol Biomarkers Prev. 2007;16:2594–604.
64. Bailey E, Erwin D, Belin P. Using cultural beliefs and patterns to improve mammography utilization among African American women: the witness project. J Natl Med Assoc. 2000;92:136–42.
65. Nigenda G, Caballero M, González-Robledo LM. Barreras de acceso al diagnóstico temprano del cáncer de mama en el Distrito Federal y en Oaxaca. Salud Publica Mex. 2009;51(Supl 2):S254–62.
66. Visvanathan K, Chlebowski RT, Hurley P, et al. American society of clinical oncology clinical practice guideline update on the Use of pharmacologic interventions including tamoxifen, raloxifene, and aromatase inhibition for breast cancer risk reduction. J Clin Oncol. 2009;27(19):3235–58.
67. Cuzick J, Forbes JF, Sestak I, et al. Long-term results of tamoxifen prophylaxis for breast cancer- 96-month follow-up of the randomized IBIS-I trial. J Natl Cancer Inst. 2007;99(4):272–82.
68. Vogel VG, Costantino JP, Wickerham DL, et al. Effects of tamoxifen vs raloxifene on the risk of developing invasive breast cancer and other disease outcomes: the NSABP Study of Tamoxifen and Raloxifene (STAR) P-2 trial. JAMA. 2006;295(23): 2727–41.
69. Hartmann LC, Schaid DJ, Woods JE, et al. Efficacy of bilateral prophylactic mastectomy in women with a family history of breast cancer. N Engl J Med. 1999;340(2):77–84.
70. Hartmann LC, Sellers TA, Schaid DJ, et al. Efficacy of bilateral prophylactic mastectomy in *BRCA1* and *BRCA2* gene mutation carriers. J Natl Cancer Inst. 2001;93(21):1633–7.
71. Rebbeck TR, Lynch HT, Neuhausen SL, et al. Prophylactic oophorectomy in carriers of *BRCA1* or *BRCA2* mutations. N Engl J Med. 2002;346(21): 1616–22.
72. Kauff ND, Satagopan JM, Robson ME, et al. Risk-reducing salpingo-oophorectomy in women with a *BRCA1* or *BRCA2* mutation. N Engl J Med. 2002; 346(21):1609–15.
73. Levine P, Veneroso C. Epidemiology of inflammatory of breast cancer. Semin Oncol. 2008;35(1):11–6.

Pathology of Inflammatory Breast Cancer

3

Victor Manuel Perez-Sanchez, Hector Aquiles Maldonado-Martinez, Paula Juarez-Sanchez, and Abelardo Meneses-Garcia

Introduction

Inflammatory breast cancer (IBC) remains the most aggressive and enigmatic form of invasive breast cancer (BC). The features of IBC were described nearly a century ago. Sir Charles Bell is credited with publishing the first description of inflammatory breast carcinoma (IBC) in 1807 [1]. The term "inflammatory carcinoma of the breast" was first introduced in 1924 by Lee and Tannenbaum, who provided the first comprehensive description of IBC based on their assessment of 28 patients [2].

In 1956, Haagensen [3] described the clinical characteristics that justified the designation of the disease as "inflammatory." The characteristics included rapid enlargement of the breast, generalized induration in the presence or absence of a distinct breast mass, acute manifestation of redness (erythema that must involve more than one-third of the breast), heat, edema of the skin of the breast, orange-peel appearance of skin (*peau d'orange*), diffuse and/or ill-defined swelling, and sometimes accompanying pain and tenderness within the breast and axilla.

The diagnosis of IBC is primarily clinical, although a pathological confirmation of invasive cancer is required. The most widely used definition of IBC is that which has been put forward by the American Joint Committee on Cancer (AJCC) [4]; this definition states in part that IBC is "a clinicopathologic entity characterized by diffuse erythema and edema of the breast, often without an underlying palpable mass."

Historically, IBC was a uniformly fatal disease. A major advance of the last three decades has been the introduction of a multidisciplinary approach to the management of this aggressive disease that incorporates preoperative chemotherapy, surgery, and radiation therapy. As a result, survival outcomes have improved significantly, with reports of 15-year survival rates of 20–30% [5, 6]. However, despite this progress, most women in whom IBC is diagnosed eventually experience a recurrence and die from the disease. Therefore, the current research is focused on the following objectives [7]: (a) refining the clinical diagnostic parameters to decrease subjectivity; (b) delineating diagnostic markers to enhance diagnostic accuracy; (c) developing predictive and prognostic markers to aid in treatment planning; (d) characterizing IBC at the molecular

V.M. Perez-Sanchez, M.D. • H.A. Maldonado-Martinez, M.D., Ph.D.
Department of Pathology, Instituto Nacional de Cancerologia-Mexico, Mexico City, DF, Mexico
e-mail: arzhaus@yahoo.com

P. Juarez-Sanchez, M.D.
Department of Pathology, Instituto Nacional de Cancerologia-Mexico (INCan), Ssa, Mexico City, DF, Mexico
e-mail: pesv2003@yahoo.com.mx

A. Meneses-Garcia, M.D., Ph.D. (✉)
Department of Medical Direction, Instituto Nacional de Cancerologia-Mexico, Ave. San Fernando 22, Tlalpan, Mexico City, DF, 14080, Mexico
e-mail: aameneses@hotmail.com

J.G. de la Garza-Salazar et al. (eds.), *Inflammatory Breast Cancer*,
DOI 10.1007/978-0-85729-991-8_3, © Springer-Verlag London 2013

level; and (e) developing targeted therapies based on an enhanced understanding of the biology of IBC, with the hope that such an approach will positively impact prognostic outcomes.

In this chapter, we review the pathological characteristics, conventional biomarkers, other biological factors, the role of stem cells, and the molecular classification of IBC.

The Biopsy

When performing a skin biopsy, in order to increase the chance of detecting dermal lymphatic involvement, it is best to sample the most prominent area of discoloration. A small skin-punch biopsy device can be used one or more times and can obtain tissue cores that range from 2 to 8 mm in diameter. This has provided sufficient tissue for determining the histology, tumor grade, hormonal receptors, monoclonal antibodies, and the presence or absence of tumor emboli in the dermis.

Macroscopic Pathology

The breast can be diffusely involved, and the size and distribution of the primary tumors are difficult to obtain. Most carcinomas are central in location and occupy virtually the entire breast [8]. The redness of the skin, which is the most distinctive clinical feature of IBC, is not always visible in excised specimens. Evaluation of skin margins is not practical since dermal lymphatic involvement cannot be noted grossly, such as the redness, and is usually less evident in excised specimens. Thickening of the skin is usually significant and secondary to dermal fibrosis. Cutaneous ulceration is not common, although nipple retraction is common in patients with IBC [9].

The breast parenchyma may appear nearly normal in many patients who have a complete pathological response (cPR). Tumors within the breast parenchyma after neoadjuvant chemotherapy can grossly resemble scar tissue, although visible gross tumors are frequently not evident [9].

Histological Findings

The signs of inflammation are a manifestation of an extensive dermal lymphatic invasion by cancer cells. The disease, primarily a continuous growth of carcinoma through the lymphatic vessels, is essentially a subepidermal carcinomatous lymphatic permeation that eventually blocks the entire lymphatic and venous plexus. Many of the vascular spaces that contain tumor cells are considered lymphatics, but tumor cells can also be present in blood vessels. Figures 3.1 and 3.2 show tumor emboli of IBC. Intradermal invasive carcinoma is not a typical feature of IBC at presentation but can occur as the disease advances. Any changes, whether rare or moderately common, which are caused by true inflammation, as indicated by the infiltration of lymphocytes and monocytes, will be evident mainly in perivascular areas; inflammation is a response to lymphatic blockage by cancer cells. Neutrophils, eosinophils, and mast cells are not common in IBC [9].

Despite adequate sampling of the skin, including evaluation of multiple levels of the tissue block, dermal tumor emboli may be identified in not more than 75 % of patients with the clinical manifestations of IBC [10, 11]. Therefore, whereas the presence of dermal lymphovascular tumor emboli is useful in confirming the clinical diagnosis of IBC, their absence does not negate a diagnosis of IBC in patients who present with the characteristic skin findings and demonstrate invasive carcinoma in the underlying breast [12].

The breast skin of patients with IBC often displays a variety of histologic alterations, such as a broader-than-normal collagenous reticular dermal layer, which is a result of increased collagen and edema. Lymphatic dilation tends to be prominent in the papillary and reticular dermis, and scattered tumor emboli can become evident at either level of the dermis. Lymphatic tumor emboli can be detected in areas that appear to be clinically uninvolved.

IBC is not related to any specific histologic type of carcinoma of the breast [8, 13–15]. IBC presentation has usually been associated with invasive ductal carcinoma that is nearly always poorly

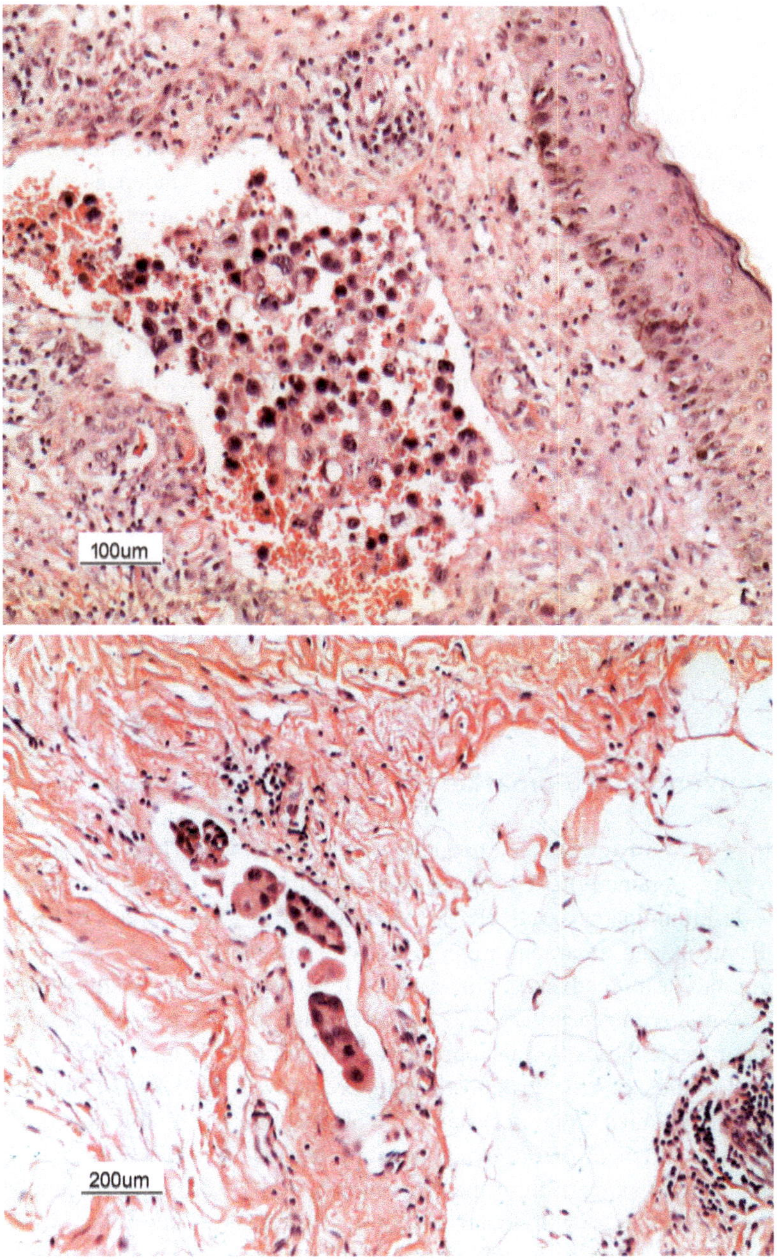

Figs. 3.1 and 3.2 Tumor emboli of inflammatory breast cancer (*IBC*), H&E stain (Fig. 3.1 200x, Fig. 3.2 100x)

differentiated, but it also has been associated with invasive lobular carcinoma, medullary carcinoma, colloid carcinoma, and comedo-type ductal carcinoma in situ. Some authors have reported that carcinoma associated with IBC is frequently multicentric and displays at least a focally micropapillary architectural pattern and extensive peritumoral lymphatic invasion [9].

Evaluation of skin margins in surgically excised specimens may not be useful because of the possibility of finding emboli in grossly unremarkable skin as well as in the skin beyond the extent of the invasive tumor in the breast.

The frequency of involvement of axillary and supraclavicular lymph nodes in different studies of patients with IBC has ranged from 60 to 85 % [16].

Differential Diagnosis

The main differential diagnosis in young women is mastitis, acute inflammation of the breast. On microscopic examination, samples from these breasts show cellular detritus and true inflammatory changes. Other conditions in the differential diagnosis include:

1. Soft tissue sarcomas
2. Primary lymphoma of the breast
3. Secondary Hodgkin lymphoma in breast
4. In rare cases, inflammatory metastatic melanoma

This is because the mechanism of involvement in lymphoma and metastatic melanoma is similar, with multiplying malignant cells spreading through the lymphatics and causing diffuse lymphatic blockage. A biopsy and immunohistochemical studies are usually sufficient for confirming diagnosis.

Conventional Biomarkers

It is currently necessary to analyze all of the results obtained in T4 breast cancer tumors (non-inflammatory and IBC). Alternatives in diagnosis and treatment are constantly expanding, but despite advances, the rates of local and systemic recurrence vary, and it is necessary to incorporate these after an appropriate validation and studies of true prognostic and predictive value (see AJCC staging system) and others that are more relevant: *HER2/neu* gene amplification and protein expression of the other members of the epithelial growth factor receptor (EGFR) family; S-phase fraction; DNA ploidy; *p53* gene mutations; cyclin E, p27 deregulation; the presence of tumor cells in the circulation; or bone marrow perineural and/or lymphovascular space invasion.

(a) Hormonal Receptors:

Estrogen and progesterone receptors are weak prognostic markers of outcome [17] and strong predictive markers of response to endocrine therapy [18]. Estrogen receptor (ER) expression has been considered to be present in two-thirds of breast cancers [18], but recent studies suggest that its incidence may be closer to 70 % [19]. Analysis of progesterone receptor (PR) expression is reported along with ER expression. PR status is independently associated with disease-free survival (DFS) and overall survival (OS); that is, patients with ER-positive/PR-positive tumors have a better prognosis than patients with ER-positive/PR-negative tumors, who in turn have a better prognosis than patients with ER-negative/PR-negative tumors [20].

IBC has a negative ER and PR status more frequently than non-IBC. Up to 55–83 % of IBC tumors are negative compared with other forms of locally advanced breast cancer (LABC) [21]. Paradiso et al. determined the level of cytosolic ER and PR in IBC compared with LABC and found ER and PR positivity in 44 and 30 %, respectively, of IBC versus 64 and 51 % of LABC [22]. Patients with ER-negative tumors had a median survival of 2 years compared with 4 years in patients with ER-positive tumors. Somlo et al. reported better relapse-free survival (RFS) in patients with ER-positive IBC than in patients with ER-negative IBC [23].

Lack of ER expression is one of the parameters that belong to the IBC immunophenotypic signature [21]. Figures 3.3 and 3.4 show tumor emboli in IBC positive for ER and PR, respectively.

(b) ERBB Family:

EGFR and its close relatives HER2/cERBB2, ERBB3, and ERBB4 are type 1 transmembrane receptor tyrosine kinases (RTK) with key roles in embryonic development, tissue renewal/repair, and cancer. A great deal has been learned about their structure, signaling pathways, and aberrations linked to malignant transformation since the explosion of interest in this family in the 1980s [24].

Although HER2 overexpression and/or amplification rates have been reported in up to 100 % of IBC tumors tested [25], the most common rate is close to 40–50 % of IBC overexpressing HER2 [21]. The differences in HER2 status between IBC and non-IBC

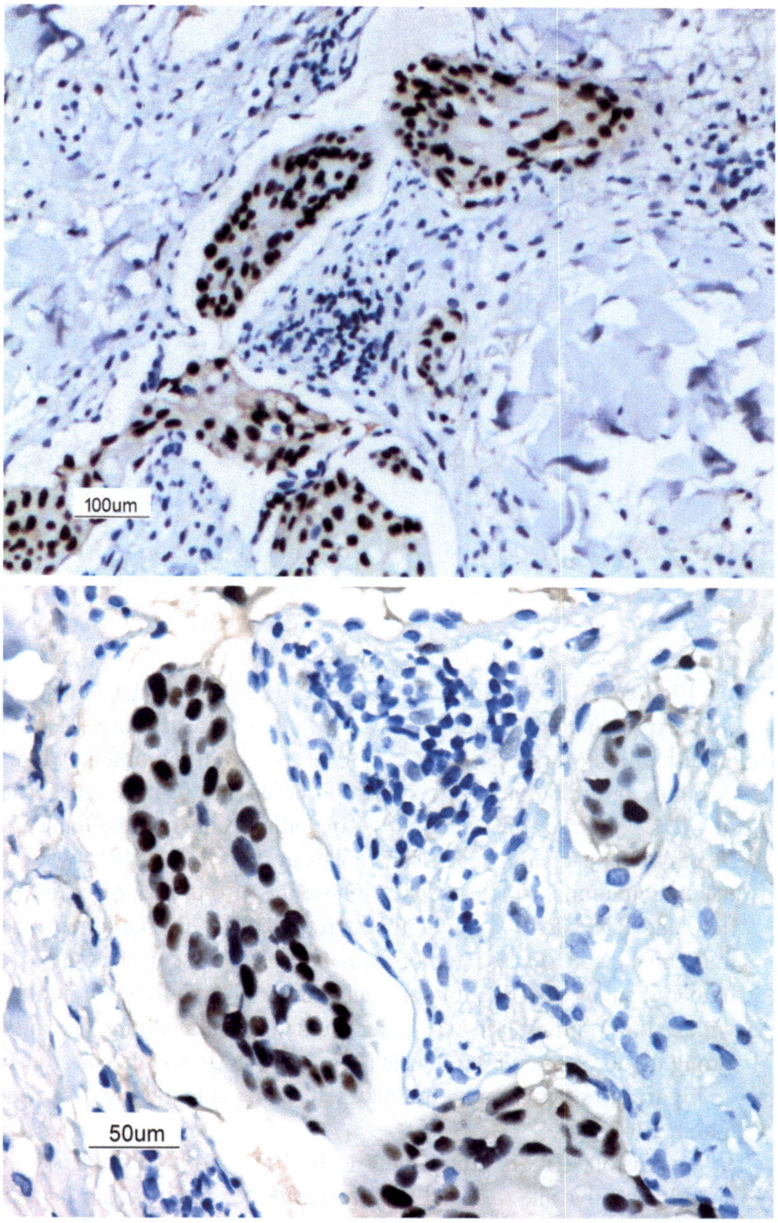

Figs. 3.3 and 3.4 Tumor emboli in inflammatory breast cancer (*IBC*) positive for estrogen receptor (*ER*) and progesterone receptor (*PR*), respectively (Fig. 3.3 200x, Fig. 3.4 400x)

have been observed at the molecular level, with IBC tumors more frequently showing gene amplification (by Southern blotting) and mRNA expression (by Northern blotting, RT-PCR) compared with non-IBC tumors. These observations indicate that HER2-directed therapy may improve survival in patients with IBC [25].

IBC has a higher incidence of EGFR and HER2 overexpression than non-IBC. Le et al. reported that patients with IBC were not often associated with lack of hormonal receptors but rather were associated with a positive expression of EGFR (58 %) and HER2 (60 %) [26]. A study with 225 patients with LABC including IBC revealed that EGFR expression is an independent adverse prognostic factor, particularly when coexpressed with HER2 [27]. This result largely suggested the potential benefit of dual EGFR/ERBB2 targeting.

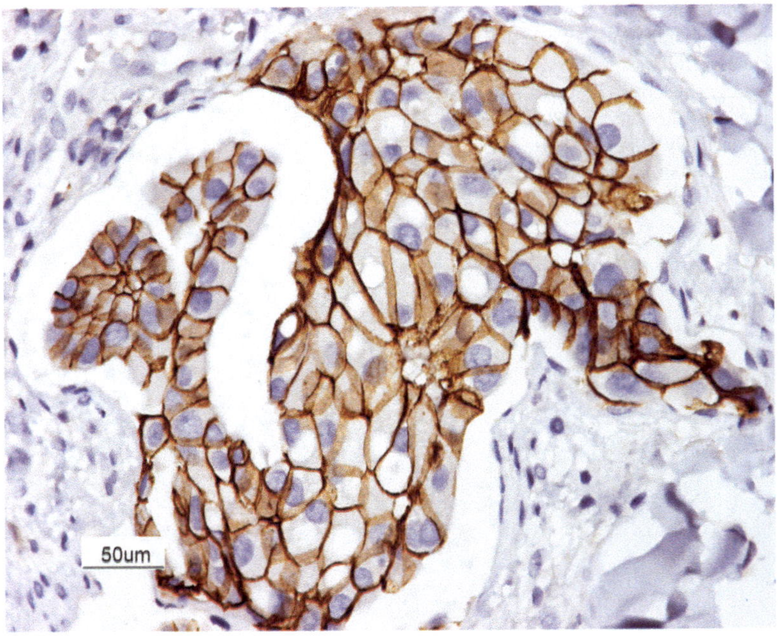

Fig. 3.5 Tumor emboli of inflammatory breast cancer (*IBC*) overexpressing HER2/neu (400×)

Figure 3.5 shows tumor emboli of IBC overexpressing HER2/neu.

(c) Proliferation Markers:

A higher proliferation rate has been observed in IBC by several methods, including 3 H-thymidine labeling index, Ki67 index evaluated by immunohistochemistry, S-phase fraction, and RT-PCR. In a study, it was reported that cell kinetics in IBC tumors was twofold higher than in non-IBC tumors, and tumors with a low proliferation rate demonstrated a strong trend for a better prognosis [22].

Figure 3.6 shows tumor emboli of IBC with a high KI67 index.

In conclusion, IBC is more likely to be ER- and PR-negative and to have EGFR and HER2 overexpression and a more rapid growth rate than non-IBC.

Novel Molecular Targets

Angiogenesis

Research on tumor angiogenesis is a major focus in biomedicine. Vasculogenesis and angiogenesis are two distinct processes. The former represents vessel formation from differentiated precursors, while the latter originates from the preexisting vasculature. Angiogenesis is essential during development, while in adulthood, the vasculature is usually quiescent, except during wound healing and the female reproductive cycle [28].

Dr. Virchow was the first to identify a huge number of blood vessels in tumors in 1863. In 1907, Goldman was the first to describe tumor vascularization in carcinomas of the stomach, the liver, and other organs. Murphy reported concerning the angiogenic response induced by Jensen rat sarcoma cells in chick chorioallantoic membrane (CAM) in 1913. The term "angiogenesis" was first used in 1935 and described the formation of new blood vessels in the placenta and, 4 years later, in wound healing and tumor growth [29]. However, it was not until 1971 that Folkman proposed that tumor growth and metastasis depend on angiogenesis and that inhibition of angiogenesis may be a potential way to inhibit cancer progression. He hypothesized that a tumor would remain in dormancy at a microscopic size (1–2 mm) in the absence of angiogenesis [30]. Subsequently, independent studies by Senger and Dvorak, Ferrara and Henzel, as well as Connolly and colleagues led to the purification, identification, and cloning of the vascular endothelial growth factor (VEGF),

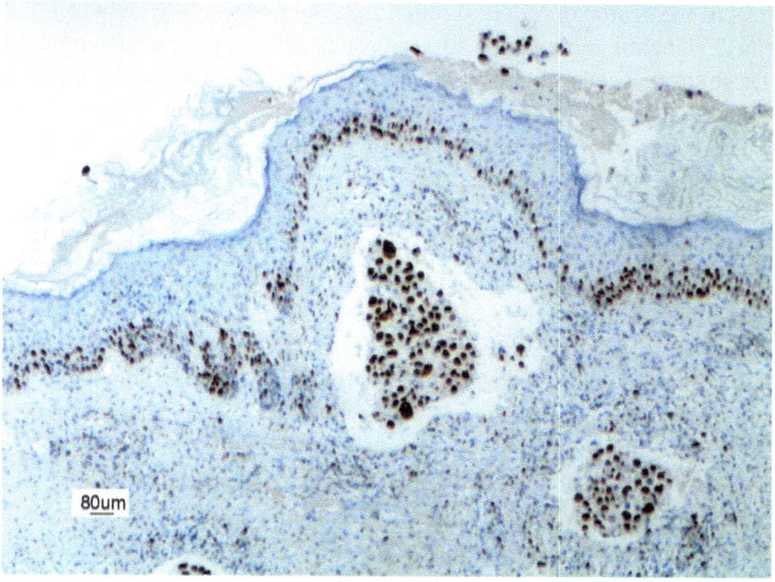

Fig. 3.6 Tumor emboli of inflammatory breast cancer (*IBC*) with a high KI67 index (60×)

the key proangiogenic factor [29]. Since then, our knowledge of molecular mechanisms to tumor angiogenesis has continually increased, leading to the discovery of promising antiangiogenic therapies for patients with tumors.

In fact, all mammalian cells, including tumor cells, are restricted to within 100–200 μm of a capillary blood vessel due to an oxygen diffusion limit at about 100 μm [31].

During tumorigenesis, the appropriate balance between pro- and antiangiogenic molecules is lost, with the balance skewed toward a proangiogenic phenotype driven by the acquisition by tumor cells of properties required for their unopposed growth. The angiogenic switch, a rapid increase of blood vessel formation to support tumor growth, is triggered by the following: (1) oncogene-mediated tumor expression of angiogenic proteins including VEGF, fibroblast growth factor (FGF), platelet-derived growth factor (PDGF), EGF, lysophosphatic acid (LPA), and angiopoietin (Ang); (2) metabolic and/or mechanical stress; (3) genetic mutations; (4) the immune response; and perhaps most prominently (5) hypoxia [29].

Because tumor cells are in a hypoxic state prior to the angiogenic switch, the HIF1 pathway is constitutively active and leads to the expression of angiogenesis-related genes (*VEGF/VEGFR*, *MMP*, *Eph/ephrin*), which greatly contribute to VEGF production. VEGFs amplify this system through the VEGF-dependent matrix metalloproteinase (MMP) expression involved in extracellular matrix (ECM) degradation and growth factor release [28]. VEGF acts in combination with nitric oxide (NO) to increase vessel permeability in order to allow extravasation of the plasma proteins needed to facilitate endothelial cell (EC) migration [28]. VEGF stimulation also mediates VEGF receptor (VEGFR) activation for proteinase expression and vascular endothelial-cadherin (VE-CAD) complex disruption, leading to endothelial cell/cell and cell/matrix detachment. During this process, parallel stimulation of Tie2 by Ang2 induces pericyte detachment. Endothelial cell detachment is required for endothelial cell migration and proliferation [29]. VEGF then triggers vessel sprouting, working as chemoattractant on endothelial detaching cells from the nearest vessels. Coordinated production of VEGF stimulates VEGFR2 expression at the tip cells in the sprout and, through VEGFR1 upregulation, leads to the expression of Dll4 in stalk cells (cells in the sprout immediately behind tips cells). Dll4 is a NOTCH ligand that inhibits the transformation of stalk cells into tip cells. In this way, tip cells lead the sprout, while stalk cells proliferate to elongate the neovessel and create a lumen in it [28]. While tip cells drive vessel elongation toward the source of VEGF through EphB4/ephrinB2 signaling, tumor cells attract stromal cells. These stromal cells, comprising tumor-associated macrophages and fibroblasts, contribute to tumor angiogenesis through the secretion of proangiogenic factors [28, 32]. During vessel elongation, new ECM is synthesized, and a few pericytes will cover the neovessel [32]. This, in conjunction with NO production and disruption of the adherens junction, results in a leaky neovessel. It is important to emphasize that the resulting vasculature in malignant neoplasms is not normal; it is composed of leaky, tortuous vessels with many dead ends, prone to cell extravasation. Moreover, endothelial cells in these vessels contribute to tumor growth by secreting supporting molecules in addition to carrying nutrients and oxygen.

In addition to supporting tumor growth, angiogenesis facilitates metastasis. The structurally abnormal newly formed tumor blood vessels with increased numbers of fenestrations, vesicles, and vesicovacuolar channels and the lack of normal basement membrane are more permeative and would constitute the easier entry point for tumor cells into the circulation, hence promoting distant metastases [32].

VEGF expression is upregulated in breast cancer. VEGF production and secretion within the breast cancer microenvironment is triggered by a number of stimuli including growth factors, cytokines, hormones, loss of *p53* function, *RAS* and *SRC* mutations, and hypoxia, as well as overexpression of HER2 (HER2/neu, ERBB2). Moreover, high levels of MMP-9 are produced and secreted by BC cells and release sequestered VEGF from the adjacent ECM. Importantly, VEGF levels are higher in premenopausal than in postmenopausal patients, indicating that steroid hormones increase VEGF expression [29].

Indeed, upregulation of VEGF in tumor cell lines is triggered by the interaction of the ERα/estradiol complex with an imperfect estrogen response element located 1.5 kb upstream of the VEGF transcription start site [29].

Another regulator of angiogenesis in breast cancer is osteoprotegerin (OPG), a glycoprotein belonging to the TNF receptor (TNFR) superfamily whose production is triggered by direct cell-EC contact [33]. High levels of OPG are present in tumor EC and correlate with tumor grade in breast cancer [34]. Similarly, the transcription factor HOXB9 is overexpressed in 42 % of patients with BC. It induces production of transforming growth factor beta (TGFβ), ERBB ligands, and several angiogenic factors (VEGF, βFGF, IL-8, and ANGPTL-2), thereby resulting in the induction of mesenchymal cell fate, invasion, as well as angiogenesis [35].

The *FES* proto-oncogene (also known as *FPS*), which encodes an SRC homology 2 (SH2) domain-containing cytoplasmic protein tyrosine kinase (PTK), mediates tumor angiogenesis and metastasis [36]. Indeed, the tumor microenvironment in *fes*-deficient mice showed reduced vascularity and fewer tumor-associated macrophages, indicating a therapeutic role for *FES* inhibition [37].

Assessment of Tumor Vascularity in Breast Cancer

The classical paper of Weidner et al. demonstrated that by immunostaining the blood vessels, the number of microvessels per 200× field in the highest neovascularization areas (hotspots) correlated with distant metastasis in patients with breast cancer, corresponding to a 1.17-fold (95 % confidence interval [95 % CI] = 1.02–1.34) increase in the distant metastasis risk for every increase in ten microvessels [38]. Among the commonly used antibodies are antibodies against factor-VIII-related antigens CD31 and CD34. Anti-CD34 is now considered the optimal marker due to its higher sensitivity without high failure rate in antigen retrieval for invasive breast carcinoma.

Another factor to consider in assessing microvessel density is the variation from the original method designed by Weidner et al. This includes variables such as the number of hotspots counted, the areas and fields of magnification (magnification of a field area of 200× or 400×), the subjectivity in identification of what constitutes a stained blood vessel, and also the descriptive statistics in reporting the number of microvessel density (the mean or the highest value). To overcome observer subjectivity, a 25-point Chalkley microscope eyepiece graticule has been introduced. The graticule is orientated in such a way that it gives the maximum number of graticule points overlapping the highlighted vessels. This method measures relative area and has strong association with vessel area and number [39]. Both the conventional optical assessment method and the Chalkley method have been used in studies that demonstrated increased microvessel density as a poor prognostic factor. Controversies over the best methodology remain despite a proposed consensus of using the Chalkley method in angiogenesis quantification in solid human tumors.

Vessel Formation in Inflammatory Breast Cancer

Consistent with its aggressive phenotype, IBC shows increased vessel numbers in comparison with non-IBC. McCarthy et al. evaluated microvessel density (MVD) using the Weidner method with antibodies directed at CD31 and found this to be significantly higher in IBC (25.5 microvessels per 400× field) than in non-IBC (6.5 microvessels per 400× field) samples [40]. A different study using the Chalkey method corroborates this finding and demonstrates higher proliferation fraction of endothelial cells in IBC (15 %) when compared with non-IBC, as well as higher proportion of immature endothelial cells (90 %) in IBC [41].

The greater vascularity in IBC correlates with angiogenic processes in IBC. In support of this, Auwera et al. using quantitative PCR, reported that IBC specimens have shown, in comparison with non-IBC samples, significantly higher mRNA expression levels of different proangiogenic mediators such as angiopoietin-1, Tie-1, Tie-2, βFGF, and COX2. COX2 and βFGF have also shown increased expression at the protein level by immunohistochemistry [41, 42]. Discordant results for VEGF and angiopoietin-2 have been recorded by two different studies: while Auwera et al. found no differences in the expression of this to genes between IBC and non-IBC samples, Bieche et al. found significant differences among these two groups [41, 43]. In a similar manner, lymphangiogenesis is increased in IBC. Levels of mRNA of the genes coding for lymphangiogenic factors such as *VEGFC VEGFD*, their receptor *VEGFR3*, and lymphatic endothelial markers PROX-1 and LYVE-1 were found to be significantly (*all p* values <0.02) higher in IBC in contrast to non-IBC [41, 42].

In addition to angio- and lymphangiogenic activity in IBC, alternative pathways have been proposed for vessel, tumor emboli, and metastasis formation in this subset of tumors. For instance, it has been demonstrated that in IBC as well as in other neoplasms such as melanoma, the tumor cells themselves act as EC to form functional avascular blood conduits or mosaic blood vessels. This process has been called "vasculogenic mimicry" and has been proposed to explain the lack of necrosis in IBC tumoral nests in comparison to non-IBC, at least in murine models under both conditions [44]. With respect to tumor emboli formation in IBC, which is characteristically extensive, this has been proposed by different groups as resulting from endothelial encircling of tumor nests rather than tumor cell invasion of vessels. In this process, endothelial cells would entirely surround small tumor nests, making them enter into the vessel and the circulation [45], ultimately resulting in distant metastasis [46]. Indeed, this has been demonstrated by one of these same study groups to constitute a pathway for metastasis in animal models generated with selected cell lines [45, 46].

Role of the Adhesion Molecules

Several studies have investigated the molecular mechanism associated with the characteristic histopathologic features of IBC. It has been proposed that the molecular basis of dermal lymphatic invasion might involve adhesion molecules (either on tumor cells or on endothelial cells) or angiogenic growth factors and proteolytic enzymes elaborated by tumor cells that enable intravasation.

E-cadherin is a calcium-dependent transmembrane glycoprotein that, as part of a membrane complex with α-catenin, β-catenin, and actin cytoskeleton, is essential for maintaining adhesion among epithelial cells [25]. In the majority of epithelial malignancies, including breast carcinoma,

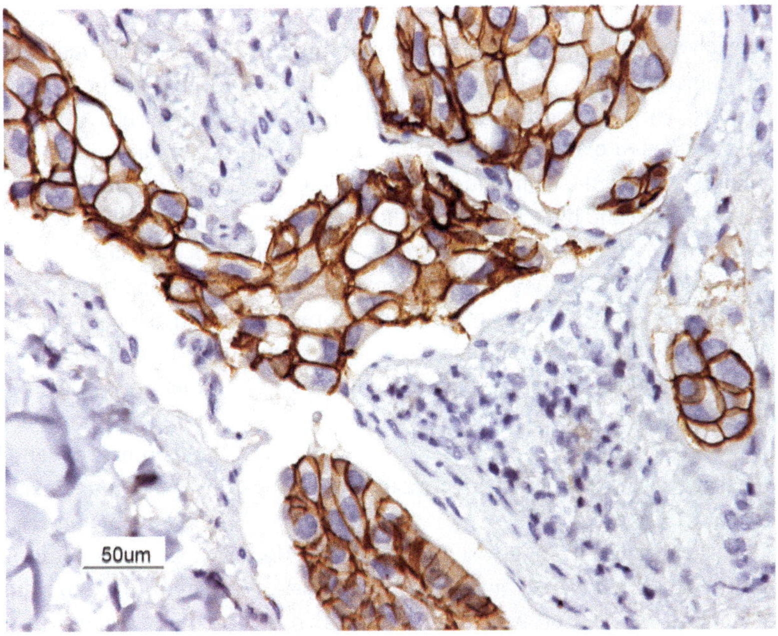

Fig. 3.7 Tumor emboli of inflammatory breast cancer (*IBC*)-diffuse E-cadherin expression evidenced by immunohistochemistry (400×)

decreased or lost E-cadherin expression is associated with malignant progression: high histologic grade, increased proliferation, invasion, metastasis, and poor prognosis [25, 47]. E-cadherin is thought to be a tumor suppressor because cancer cells must break intercell adhesions before attaining a motile phenotype [48]. Paradoxically, however, an up to 10–20-fold overexpression of E-cadherin was found in an IBC xenograft model (MARY-X) in comparison with non-IBC cell lines and xenografts [49, 50]. Other reports have shown that higher E-cadherin expression was also observed in a human IBC cell line (SUM149) rather than in a non-IBC cell line (SUM102) [51]. Immunohistochemical study of 20 IBC and 22 stage-matched non-IBC tumors showed that E-cadherin was preferentially expressed in IBC tumors (100 % IBC vs. 68 % non-IBC). No association was found between E-cadherin expression and hormonal receptors or HER2 status [52]. Similarly, Colpaert et al. reported strong E-cadherin expression in 33 of 35 IBC tumors. In particular, intralymphatic tumor emboli of IBC strongly expressed E-cadherin. Figure 3.7 shows tumor emboli of IBC diffuse E-cadherin expression evidenced by immunohistochemistry.

Immunohistochemical findings suggested that E-cadherin is required for formation of tumor emboli and acts by enhancing tumor cell-tumor cell adhesion and maintaining the integrity of IBC tumor emboli in the dermal lymphatics. Such cohesive tumor aggregates may provide a survival benefit [53]. Previous studies suggested that tumor cell emboli are more efficient at forming metastases than single cells and that tumor cell emboli are hypoxic in their centers and are therefore more resistant to chemotherapy and radiation therapy than single cells [54].

Intravasation of tumor cells into lymphatic vessels is the initial step for lymphatic metastasis. The tightly bound tumor cells may be passively disseminated into newly formed vascular channels around them [55]. It also has been postulated that E-cadherin expression varies at different stages of the disease and that it is transiently lost during tumor invasion into lymphovascular channels and reinstates its expression once tumor cells intravasate into the circulation [52].

Studies focused on E-cadherin as a potential therapeutic target have demonstrated that blockade of E-cadherin by using anti-E-cadherin antibodies results in loss of homotypic aggregation of MARY-X spheroids in vitro. Intravenous (i.v.) anti-E-cadherin antibodies in animals bearing MARY-X tumors with known pulmonary

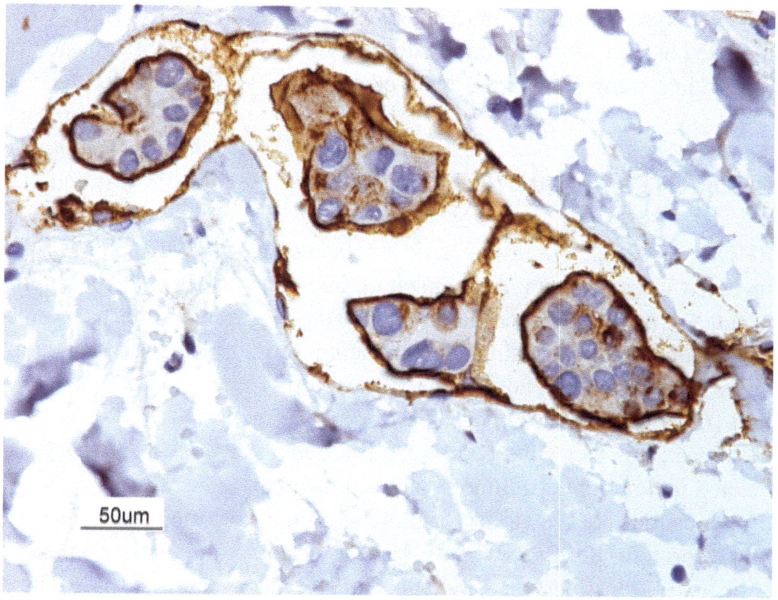

Fig. 3.8 Tumor emboli of inflammatory breast cancer (*IBC*) with patchy-cytoplasmic MUC 1 expression evidenced by immunohistochemistry (400×)

metastasis induced dissolution of the metastatic lesions. In vitro, mutant MARY-X spheroids with a dominant-negative E-cadherin phenotype (H-2 K[d]-E-cad) lacking the extracellular binding domain but retaining the β-catenin binding domain similarly resulted in loss of homotypic aggregation. In mice, these dominant-negative mutant constructs were only weakly tumorigenic and did not form tumor emboli [50, 56].

Other studies using the SUM149 IBC cell line demonstrated that the presence of dominant-negative E-cadherin (H-2kd-E-cad) cDNA blocked the robust invasion of SUM149 cells in vitro, which was associated with decreased expression of the matrix metalloproteinase (MMP) enzymes MMP-1 and MMP-9. These studies suggest that the process of invasion and intravasation by IBC tumor emboli was mediated by both E-cadherin and enhanced proteolytic enzyme activity [57]. In support of the role of E-cadherin and related molecules in IBC, there are recent studies demonstrating that blockade of p120-catenin, which anchors E-cadherin, or inhibition of the translation initiation factor eIF4GI, which regulates translation of specific mRNAs such as p120, results in loss of integrity of SUM149 tumor spheroids [58]. These findings collectively suggest that the E-cadherin molecule is central to the intravasation of IBC tumor emboli and represents an important target for effective treatment of IBC.

In addition to an intact and overexpressed E-cadherin/α,β-catenin axis, sialyl-Lewis X/A-deficient mucin 1 (MUC1) appears to be another key factor that contributes to lymphovascular metastasis of IBC [55, 59]. MUC1 is a glycoprotein in the cell surface mucin family and the ligand of E-selectin (a cell adhesion receptor) on the surface of endothelial cells. The sialyl-Lewis X/A carbohydrate ligand-binding epitope on MUC1 facilitates ligand-receptor interaction [55]. Nonsialylated MUC1 does not bind to E-selectin, resulting in epithelial cell-endothelial cell aversion. Alpaugh et al. demonstrated that MARY-X spheroid cells expressed the sialyl-Lewis X/A-deficient MUC1 because of decreased α3/4-fucosyltransferase activity, which leads to lack of binding of tumor cells to endothelial cells and facilitates dissemination of tumor emboli [55, 59]. The increased cytoplasmic MUC1 found in IBC with immunohistochemistry could reflect the accumulation of this "nonfunctional" MUC1. Taken together, overexpression of E-cadherin and dysfunctional MUC1 may cooperate synergistically to contribute to the highly metastatic phenotype of IBC. Figure 3.8 shows tumor emboli of IBC with patchy-cytoplasmic MUC 1 expression evidenced by immunohistochemistry.

Overexpression of E-cadherin and MUC1 was included as part of the "inflammatory signature" of IBC in a study by Charafe-Jauffret et al. [25].

RHOC GTPase and WISP3

RHOC GTPase, a breast-specific oncogene, is involved in cytoskeletal reorganization and contributes to metastatic potential by increasing cellular motility and invasion, and inducing actin stress fiber and focal adhesion complex formation [60]. *WISP3* is a tumor-suppressor gene in the breast; it is located at 6q22-q23, a frequently deleted region in breast tumors, and is a member of the insulin-like growth factor-binding protein-related protein (IGFBP-rP) family [61, 62]. These two genes were identified by Van Golen et al. [61] and contribute to the highly invasive phenotype of IBC. With in situ hybridization, *RHOC* guanosine triphosphatase (GTPase) was found to be overexpressed in 90 % of IBC tumors compared with 38 % of stage-matched non-IBC tumors, whereas *WISP3* (also known as "lost in inflammatory breast cancer" or *LIBC*) was lost in 80 % of IBC tumors versus in only 21 % of non-IBC tumors. Kleer et al. [63, 64] found that *RHOC* overexpression was associated with high histologic grade, positive lymph node status, and negative hormonal receptor status and HER2 overexpression. In addition, high *RHOC* expression was shown to be a predictor of poor OS in patients with breast cancer, as well as being an independent predictor of poor response to doxorubicin-based chemotherapy. Transfection of *RHOC* in nontransformed breast cells leads to an IBC-like phenotype with regard to invasion and motility [60]. *RHOC* overexpression in IBC is also associated with upregulation of *VEGF, βFGF, IL-6,* and *IL-8*, leading to the formation of a specific type of angiogenic stroma [65, 66].

Overexpression of WISP3 in SUM149 greatly reduced cell motility, invasion, anchorage-independent growth, and cell growth rate. Loss of WISP3 expression is hypothesized to contribute to the proliferative and invasive phenotype of IBC [62]. In vitro experiment suggested that the effect of *RHOC* may be modulated by WISP3 expression [62, 67]. Specific targeted knockdown of WISP3 in nontransformed mammary epithelial cells led to increased expression of *RHOC*, which in turn resulted in expression of invasion-related genes promoting a metastatic phenotype. WISP3-restored SUM149 cells had a significantly inhibited capacity for invasion. It appears that *RHOC* and WISP3 might act in concert to contribute to the aggressive phenotype of IBC and may serve as promising prognostic indicators and possible therapeutic targets for IBC [25].

Other Biologic Factors

Mutations in the *p53* tumor suppressor gene are the most common mutations found in human cancers [68]. Thirty percent of breast cancers contain mutations in one of the p53 alleles, and it has been demonstrated that on progression, approximately 60 % of these breast cancers lose the mutant and retain the wild-type allele [69]. Loss of function in the tumor suppressor gene *p53* (*TP53*) has been shown to contribute to the initiation of breast cancer; consequently, tumors with mutant *TP53* genes have been found to have increased cellular proliferation and a poorer overall prognosis. Mutant *TP53* occurs more frequently in IBC, which might contribute to the aggressive behavior of this disease. In addition, wild-type *TP53* might be functionally inactivated by sequestration of p53 protein within the cytoplasm, where it is unable to coordinate activity within the nucleus. This could account for the presence of wild-type p53 in IBC, yet its tumor-suppressing function remains inactive, thus governing its clinical course [70].

Analysis of 27 patients with IBC using multivariate analysis concluded a positive relationship between high levels of p53 detected in the nucleus and poor clinical outcome [71]. To correlate p53 status and prognosis, the analysis was extended by an additional group of 24 patients with IBC who were screened for *p53* mutations, p53 mRNA levels, and protein expression [72].

The patients with a *p53* gene mutation and nuclear overexpression of the p53 protein had an 8.6-fold higher risk of death compared with patients who had no mutation and no protein overexpression. Combined with ER data, risk of death increased with ER negativity. These findings regarding *p53* status and IBC were confirmed by further study, and weak association between *p53* mutation plus negative ER status and lower response rate to therapy was also apparent [73].

The nuclear transcription factor κB (NF-κB) is an important mediator of cell proliferation, apoptosis, and migration. Van Laere et al. reported significant overexpression of many NF-κB target genes in IBC tumors compared with non-IBC tumors by cDNA microarray, and this was confirmed by RT-PCR [74, 75]. Similarly, at the protein level, the amount of nuclei positively stained by immunohistochemistry for two NF-κB subunits (RelB and NF-κB1) was significantly increased in IBC and showed significant correlation with the results of NF-κB DNA-binding experiments for these same subunits [75]. These authors also found evidence for an ER-negative-mediated inhibition of the NF-κB signaling pathway since NF-κB target genes were significantly elevated in ER-negative versus ER-positive breast tumors, and the amount of immunostained nuclei for RelB and NFkB1 was higher in ER-negative versus ER-positive breast tumors [75].

Further investigation on NF-kB transcription factor activation in breast cancer in terms of ER signaling demonstrates that NF-kB activation is not exclusively limited to IBC but is more generalized in ER-negative breast tumors. However, Van Laere et al. have demonstrated that IBC is characterized by mitogen-activated protein kinase (MAPK) hyperactivation in comparison with non-IBC and that the inverse correlation between NF-kB activation and ER activation is potentially due to EGFR and/or ERBB2 overexpression with subsequent MAPK hyperactivation, resulting in NF-kB activation and ER downregulation [76].

Altogether, these findings suggest that the NF-κB transcription factor pathway plays an important role in the aggressive behavior of IBC, and targeted inhibition of NF-κB activation may offer therapeutic potential in IBC. In particular, NF-kB and MAPK might be therapeutic targets for IBC specifically and more generally for ER-negative breast tumors, as well as for breast tumors with acquired resistance to hormonal therapy [76].

Chemokine receptors and their ligands have been thought to play a role in the metastatic process of breast cancer [25]. A study suggested that the expression of chemokine receptors (CXCR4 and CCR7) was associated with an increased risk of recurrence and death in patients with IBC [77].

Studies using the SUM149 and SUM190 IBC cell lines document a role for prostaglandin-endoperoxide synthase 2, also known as cyclooxygenase-2 (COX2), in the invasive and angiogenic phenotype of IBC, which confirms previous reported results from gene expression and tissue microarray studies that were the first to identify COX2 overexpression in IBC tumors [42].

Overexpression of COX2 and elevated levels of its enzymatic product prostaglandin E2 (PGE2) is a characteristic of invasive human breast cancers and is detectable at early stages of tumorigenesis. COX2 also directly regulates the P450 Cyp191A1 aromatase enzyme, thereby regulating estrogen production, and interacts with both HER2 and EGFR. COX2 is one of a group of genes that mediate tumor extravasation, survival, and reinitiation at distant sites during metastasis [78].

The roles of COX2 and the associated PGE2 prostanoid receptor family in the metastatic phenotype of IBC are currently under active investigation and represent important therapeutic targets in IBC.

$p27^{KIP1}$ is a cyclin-dependent kinase inhibitor. The $p27^{kip1}$ deregulation manifested by low protein cellular concentration might represent an adverse prognostic marker in IBC and could provide a valuable tool for selecting treatment for this aggressive disease [79].

A summary of some of the principal molecular markers is shown in Table 3.1.

Cancer Stem Cells/Epithelial-Mesenchymal Transition

Stem cells have the capacity to self-renew and to generate daughter cells that can differentiate through several lineages to form all of the cell

Table 3.1 Molecular markers in inflammatory breast cancer: IBC versus non-IBC

Study	RHOC	HER2+	ER−	PR−	E-cadherin expression	p53 expression	LIBC/WISP3 expression	MUC1	NF-kB1/RelB expression
Nguyen [80]	NA	26 vs. 17 %	49 vs. 30 %	68 vs. 43 %	87 % vs. NA	32 vs. 52 %	NA	NA	NA
Turpin [81]	NA	36 vs. 27 %	NA	NA	NA	57 vs. 30 %	NA	NA	NA
van Golen [61]	90 vs. 38 %	NA	NA	NA	NA	NA	20 vs. 79 %	NA	NA
Ben Hamida [82]	NA	33 vs. 14 %	54 vs. 26 %	53 vs. 36 %	NA	42 vs. 30 %	NA	93 vs. 87 %	NA
Van Laere [75]	NA	NA	73 vs. 37 %	77 vs. 43 %	NA	NA	NA	NA	68 vs. 50 % (NF-kB1)
									36 vs. 0 % (RelB)
Charafe-Jauffret [83]	NA	40 vs. 12 %	54 vs. 24 %	54 vs. 35 %	44 vs. 10 %	45 vs. 23 %	NA	74 vs. 41 %	NA

IBC inflammatory breast cancer, *ER* estrogen receptor, *PR* progesterone receptor, *LIBC* lost in inflammatory breast cancer, *WISP3* WNT inducible signaling pathway protein 3, *MUC1* mucin 1 (cytoplasmic staining), *NA* not available

types that are found in mature tissue. Stem cells might undergo an asymmetric cell division, producing a novel stem cell to maintain the stem cell compartment and a cell that differentiates, via additional cell divisions, into terminally differentiated cells. The cells that form the intermediates between stem cells and terminally differentiated cells are usually referred to as progenitor cells, transit cells, or transit amplifying cells. In addition, a stem cell might divide symmetrically, resulting in two identical daughter cells. These two daughter cells can either be two stem cells (expansion of the stem cell compartment), two transit/progenitor cells (depletion of stem cell compartment), or again one stem cell and one transit/progenitor cell [84]. Physiologically, stem cells perform different functions in normal human tissue, among others, tissue renewal (e.g., bone marrow, small intestine, skin) or damage repair (e.g., satellite cells of muscle) [85]. This suggests that stem cells are present in all tissues of the human body.

Stem cells can accumulate several mutations due to high replicative potential and their long lifespan, which makes them excellent candidates for the cells-of-origin of cancer. Also, mutations might cause restricted progenitors or differentiated cells to acquire properties of cancer stem cells, such as increased self-renewal potential. Either way, cancer stem cells would be distinguished from other cancer cells by their tumorigenic potential, their ability to generate additional cancer stem cells (self-renewal), and their ability to generate phenotypically diverse nontumorigenic cancer cells with more limited proliferative potential (pluripotency) [86].

The existence of a stem cell population in the adult human mammary gland is suggested by the finding that the terminal ductal lobular units (TDLU) are monoclonal in origin. It was demonstrated that the pattern of X chromosome-linked gene inactivation is the same for all cells comprising TDLU [87]. The clonal origin of individual TDLU supports a model of adult stem cells that are distributed throughout the mammary gland [85]. The further characterization of mammary (cancer) stem cells was aided by the development of an in vitro propagation system for stem cells in suspension culture. Mammary stem cells form mammospheres in suspension culture [88]. These mammospheres are spherical cell structures that are able to survive and proliferate in the absence of attachment to an exogenous substratum. Mammospheres are highly enriched in bi- or multipotent cells, as demonstrated by the ability of single cells isolated from mammospheres to generate multilineage colonies when cultured under conditions promoting differentiation. In addition, it was demonstrated that single cells obtained from mammospheres are capable of generating secondary mammospheres, suggesting that these single cells are capable of self-renewal [89]. The development of the in vitro propagation system for mammary (cancer) stem cells has aided in their further molecular characterization by means of transcriptional profiling [88].

Al-Hajj et al. [90] first suggested the contribution of mammary stem cells to carcinogenesis in the breast. Uncultured specimens of human breast cancer cells from patients were separated into fractions that expressed different surface molecules, and then injected in immunodeficient mice. As few as two hundred CD44+/CD24– cancer cells were able to consistently form tumors, whereas injection of thousands of cancer cells that had other phenotypes failed to form tumors. These CD44+/CD24– cells were able to generate new cancer stem cells as well as cells with a distinct phenotype and lower tumorigenic potential [90].

To date, several other markers besides dual labeling with CD44 and CD24 have been used to characterize putative stem cell populations in breast cancer, including ALDH1 [91], CD133 [92], and Hoechst-dye exclusion [93, 94]. Applying these markers to human tissue samples, it was demonstrated that the presence of cancer stem cells in breast tumors is particularly associated with specific basal-like (triple-negative) carcinoma, HER2/neu carcinoma, and breast tumors with mutations in the *BRCA1* gene [84]. It has been observed that the presence of stem cells in breast tumors is associated with the occurrence of metastases, poor prognosis, and resistance to therapy and that breast cancer stem cells harbor tumor-initiating capacity [84].

Several studies have focused on the molecular characteristics of breast cancer stem cells. These studies are mainly on signal transduction pathways associated with embryonic development, such as NOTCH, WNT, hedgehog, TGFβ, and bone morphogenetic protein (BMP) signaling. These signaling pathways have repeatedly been associated with tumor progression, from the induction of a hyperproliferative phenotype to tumor cell dissemination and metastatic spread [95].

Cancer stem cells are relatively quiescent and undergo replication very slowly; thus, they are defined as label-retaining cells. This characteristic renders cancer stem cells less susceptible to the cytotoxic effects of conventional chemotherapeutic agents, which primarily target actively proliferating cells. Cancer stem cells also express cassettes of multidrug transporters responsible for the rapid efflux of lipophilic and chemotherapeutic drugs, which provide additional mechanisms for cancer stem cells to resist the effects of cytotoxic therapies used to treat the majority of breast cancers [12]. Cancer stem cells have also been shown to activate survival pathways, such as the PI3K/Akt signaling pathway, that mediate resistance to ionizing radiation [96].

The histological and biological features of IBC in combination with its poor-prognosis profile and the frequent occurrence of metastases suggest that cancer stem cells play an important role in IBC.

In a MARY-X model of IBC, tumor spheroids were found to express surface markers $CD44^{+}/CD24^{-low}$, to have ALDH-1 activity and, most uniquely, to express CD133, which is consistent with MARY-X having characteristics of cancer stem cells [97].

SUM149 IBC cells were documented to express the putative stem cell surface markers $CD44^{+}/CD24^{-low}$ and to have aldehyde dehydrogenase (ALDH-1) enzyme activity, believed to be a marker of tumor-initiating activity [98].

NOTCH1 belongs to a family of transmembrane epidermal growth factor-like receptors that regulate a series of important functions in the mammary gland, including self-renewal of stem cells. In a study of 85 IBC tumors, 47 % of the tumors showed high NOTCH1 expression [99]. Higher rates of chromosomal instability and genetic alterations have been reported in IBC compared with non-IBC tumors [25].

Further support for the potential role of cancer stem cells in the aggressive phenotype of IBC derives from observations that cancer stem cells are linked with tumor progression through their ability to undergo the process of epithelial-mesenchymal transition (EMT) [100]. This ability is regulated by transcription factors that also orchestrate critical steps of organ development during embryogenesis.

The EMT is associated with a change in cancer cells from epithelial morphology to acquisition of mesenchymal morphology with an associated gain of motility. Recent studies demonstrate that breast cancer cells that undergo EMT acquire characteristics of cancer stem cells [101].

A study demonstrated that the SUM149 IBC cell line, which expresses high levels of EGFR and undergoes EMT, was sensitive to the inhibitory effects of either EGFR small interfering RNA (siRNA) or erlotinib, an inhibitor of the EGFR tyrosine kinase. Targeting EGFR through the ERK1/2 pathway blocked SUM149 invasion in vitro; interestingly, low doses of erlotinib, which had no effect on primary tumor growth, inhibited development of pulmonary metastases [102]. These results suggest that EGFR and the associated ERK signaling pathway may be important targets in the strategy of reversing the process of EMT in IBC.

Gene Expression Profiling in IBC

During the past decade, several studies have specifically looked at expression profiling. One of the earliest publications, from Bertucci et al. in 2004, used cDNA microarrays containing approximately 8,000 genes to profile 37 IBC and 44 non-IBC prechemotherapy tumor samples. The authors made a number of important observations, including their finding of the presence of extensive transcriptional heterogeneity in IBC and their demonstration that IBC exhibited overexpression of basal, immune, and vascular gene clusters and exhibited underexpression of luminal gene clusters as compared with non-IBC tumors [103]. From 55 samples belonging to this study they derived a 109-gene signature that discriminated between the two sample types. This signature was then validated in the remainder of the samples, 26 in total, with an overall performance accuracy of 85 % [103]. Using the same data set, Bertucci et al. further demonstrated that similar to non-IBC, five molecular subtypes (defined according to the Stanford intrinsic gene set)—including luminal A, luminal B, basal, HER2-positive, and normal-like—could be demonstrated in IBC. Higher frequencies of basal and HER2-positive IBC samples were observed compared with the frequencies of these two subtypes in non-IBC samples [104].

Van Laere et al. in 2005 [74] used cDNA microarrays containing approximately 6,000 genes to profile 16 IBC and 18 non-IBC prechemotherapy samples. Using supervised analysis, the authors identified 953 genes that exhibited a 1.5-fold difference in expression between the two sample types. Of these genes, 756 (retained after the exclusion of genes related to the expression of estrogen receptor 1 and HER2) resulted in a perfect segregation of IBC and non-IBC samples [74]. Using the same data set, the investigators further identified five different molecular subtypes in the two sample sets, with the basal (37 %) and HER2-positive (13 %) subtypes representing 50 % of the IBC samples [105]. In a subsequent validation of their profile in a different group of samples (19 IBC, four of these from their previous work, and 40 non-IBC samples), using a different platform (Affymetrix technology), the investigators confirmed their initial findings with regard to segregation of IBC and non-IBC cases, identifying 26 % of the IBC samples as basal and 42 % as HER2-positive [106].

Bièche et al. used real-time polymerase chain reaction (RT-PCR) to quantify the mRNA expression level of 538 candidate genes in eight IBC and eight non-IBC samples; they demonstrated a greater than twofold change in a set of 48 genes between the two sample types [43]. The investigators further identified a three-gene signature composed of epiregulin (EREG), v-myc myelocytomatosis viral-related oncogene, and sonic hedgehog (SHH). This gene signature was shown to distinguish among three subgroups of women with IBC with different recurrence rates [43]. Neither the complete 48-gene signature for IBC versus non-IBC tumors nor the 3-gene signature for prognosis have been validated in an independent group of samples.

Nguyen et al. [80] using Affymetrix U133A microarrays, defined the expression profiles of prechemotherapy samples from 13 patients with IBC and 12 patients with stage III non-IBC. Because of considerable heterogeneity across both sample types, a robust signature could not be identified; however, the investigators were able to demonstrate a higher expression of genes associated with increases in metabolic rate, lipid signaling, and cell turnover in the IBC samples than in the non-IBC samples. They also confirmed the presence of three molecular subtypes of IBC, including luminal, HER2-positive, and basal subtypes [80].

Another group at the University of Texas and MD Anderson Cancer Center also failed to identify a gene profile that was differentially expressed between IBC and non-IBC specimens. They used Affymetrix GeneChips to analyze 82 tumor samples of newly diagnosed breast cancers (25 patients with IBC, T4d, and 57 patients without IBC, T4a-c). Their approach differed from that of previous works in that they not only compared the entire IBC and non-IBC groups, but they also separated each of these into the following three distinct clinical subtypes: ER-positive/HER2-normal, HER2-amplified, and ER-negative/HER2-normal. Thus, when expression data from all IBC with all non-IBC were compared, they found no significant differences after adjusting for multiple testing. However, when IBC and non-IBC tumors were compared by clinical subtype, significant differences emerged. On the other hand, as in previous studies, they show that IBC tumors can be divided into molecular and clinical subtypes similar to those of non-IBC [107].

The most recent study comes from the group at the National Cancer Institute in Bethesda, Maryland; these investigators used Affymetrix

U133A microarrays to profile 15 IBC samples and 35 non-IBC samples. Eighty-seven percent of the IBC samples and 23 % of the non-IBC samples were obtained postchemotherapy, and each sample was obtained via laser capture microdissection. The investigators were unable to identify a significant signature in the epithelia that could distinguish between the two sample types, but they were able to identify a stromal signature that could distinguish IBC from non-IBC [108]. They further demonstrated that the 109-gene signature originally identified by Bertucci et al. performed better in classifying IBC when the tumor stroma was used instead of the epithelial tumor cells; this finding lends evidence to the hypothesis that gene expression in the stroma contributes to the IBC phenotype [108].

In a different approach, Van der Auwera et al. explored whether altered miRNA expression plays a prominent role in defining the inflammatory breast cancer (IBC) phenotype. They used quantitative PCR technology to evaluate the expression of 384 miRNAs in 20 IBC and 50 non-IBC samples and evaluated direct miRNA targets by their pair-wise correlation to the expression levels of 10,962 messenger RNAs (mRNA). The authors further compared miRNAs identified in this way to predicted miRNA targets from TargetScan5.1. A profile of 13 miRNAs was identified whose expression levels were able to predict correctly the nature of the sample analyzed (IBC vs. non-IBC). For four miRNAs (miR-29a, miR-30b, miR-342-3p, and miR-520a-5p), correlated genes were concordant with predicted targets. The authors propose these 13 miRNAs as candidate markers for the IBC subtype [109]. No validation for this profile in an independent subset of samples has been published to date.

In summary, gene expression profiles have shown contradictory results in the unsupervised approach, although most frequently showing no segregation of IBC as a different cluster in breast cancer. Notwithstanding this fact, different signatures have been developed that allow distinction between IBC and non-IBC with fair accuracy. The most important contribution of the different studies on gene expression of IBC is probably the identification of some candidate pathways for potential targeted therapies in this subgroup of tumors, such as lipid metabolism, proliferation, molecular transport, and cell death [103]. In some pathways such as NF-κB, further studies are warranted because imbalances in ER status in the populations evaluated may explain the results obtained to date [103].

References

1. Bell JC. A system of operative surgery, founded on the basis of anatomy. London: Longman, Hurst, Rees, & Orne; 1807.
2. Lee BJ, Tannenbaum NE. Inflammatory carcinoma of the breast. Surg Gynecol Obstet. 1924;39:580.
3. Haagensen CD. Inflammatory carcinoma. In: Haegensen CD, editor. Diseases of the breast. 2nd ed. Philadelphia: Saunders; 1971. p. 576–84.
4. Green FL, Page DL, Fleming ID, et al., editors. AAJCC cancer staging manual. 6th ed. New York: Springer; 2002. p. 225–81.
5. Low J, Berman A, Steinber S, et al. Long term follow up for locally advanced and inflammatory breast cancer patients treated with multimodality therapy. J Clin Oncol. 2004;22:4065–74.
6. Ueno NT, Buzdar AU, Singletary SE, et al. Combined modality treatment of inflammatory breast carcinoma: twenty years of experience at MD Anderson Center. Cancer Chemother Pharmacol. 1997;40:321–9.
7. Dawood S, Cristofanilli M. Inflammatory breast cancer: what progress have we made? Oncology. 2011;25:3.
8. Rosen PP. Inflammatory carcinoma. In: Rosen PP, editor. Rosen's breast pathology. 2nd ed. Philadelphia: Lippincott Williams & Wilkins; 2001. p. 676–83.
9. Resetkova E. Pathologic aspects of inflammatory breast carcinoma: part 1. Histomorphology and differential diagnosis. Semin Oncol. 2008;35:25–32.
10. Bonnier P, Charpin C, Lejeune C, et al. Inflammatory carcinomas of the breast: a clinical, pathological, or a clinical and pathological definition? Int J Cancer. 1995;62:382–5.
11. Charpin C, Bonnier P, Khouzami A, et al. Inflammatory breast carcinoma: an immunohistochemical study using monoclonal anti-pHer-2/neu, pS2, cathepsin, ER and PR. Anticancer Res. 1992;12:591–7.
12. Robertson F, Bondy M, Yang E, et al. Inflammatory breast cancer. The disease, the biology, the treatment. CA Cancer J Clin. 2010;60:351–75.
13. Taylor GW, Melzer A. Inflammatory carcinoma of the breast. Am J Cancer. 1938;33:33–49.
14. Haagensen CD. Inflammatory carcinoma. In: Haagensen CD, editor. Diseases of the breast. 2nd ed. Philadelphia: Saunders; 1971. p. 576–84.
15. Salzstein S. Clinically occult inflammatory carcinoma of the breast. Cancer. 1974;34:382–8.

16. Amparo RS, Angel CD, Ana LH, et al. Inflammatory breast carcinoma: pathological and clinical entity? Breast Cancer Res Treat. 2000;64:269–73.
17. Hahnel R, Woodings T, Vivian AB. Prognostic value of estrogen receptors in primary breast cancer. Cancer. 1979;44:671–5.
18. Allred DC, Harvey JM, Berardo M, et al. Prognostic and predictive factors in breast cancer by immunohistochemical analysis. Mod Pathol. 1998; 11:155–68.
19. Nadji M, Gómez-Fernández C, Ganjei-Azar P, et al. Immunohistochemistry of estrogen and progesterone receptors reconsidered: experience with 5,993 breast cancers. Am J Clin Pathol. 2005;123:21–7.
20. Mohsin SK, Weiss H, Havighurst T, et al. Progesterone receptor by immunohistochemistry and clinical outcome in breast cancer: a validation study. Mod Pathol. 2004;17:1545–54.
21. Charafe-Jauffret E, Tarpin C, Viens P, et al. Defining the molecular biology of inflammatory breast cancer. Semin Oncol. 2008;35:41–50.
22. Paradiso A, Tomassi S, Brandi M, et al. Cell kinetics and hormonal receptor status in inflammatory breast carcinoma. Comparison with locally advanced disease. Cancer. 1989;64:1922–7.
23. Somlo G, Frankel P, Chow W, et al. Prognostic indicators and survival in patients with stage IIIB inflammatory breast carcinoma after dose-intense chemotherapy. J Clin Oncol. 2004;22:1839–48.
24. Eccles S. The epidermal growth factor receptor/Erb-B/HER family in normal and malignant breast biology. Int J Dev Biol. 2011;55:685–96. doi:10.1387/ijdb.113396se.
25. Gong Y. Pathologic aspects on inflammatory breast cancer: part 2. Biologic insights into its aggressive phenotype. Semin Oncol. 2008;35:33–40.
26. Le MG, Arriagada R, Bahi J, et al. Are risk factors for breast cancer similar in women with inflammatory breast cancer and in those with non-inflammatory breast cancer? Breast. 2006;15:355–62.
27. Nieto Y, Nawaz F, Jones RB, et al. Prognostic significance of overexpression and phosphorylation of epidermal growth factor receptor (EGFR) and the presence of truncated EFGRvIII in locoregionally advanced breast cancer. J Clin Oncol. 2007;21:4405–13.
28. Rodríguez S, Huynh-Do U. The role of PTEN in tumor angiogenesis. J Oncol. 2012;11 p. doi:10.1155/2012/141236. Article ID 141236.
29. Fan F, Schimming A, Jaeger D, et al. Targeting the tumor microenvironment: focus on angiogenesis. J Clin Oncol. 2012;16 p. doi:10.1155/2012/281261. Article ID 281261.
30. Folkman J. Tumor angiogenesis therapeutic implications. N Engl J Med. 1971;285:1182–6.
31. Torres IP, Filho M, Leunig F, et al. Noninvasive measurement of microvascular and interstitial oxygen profiles in a human tumor in SCID mice. Proc Natl Acad Sci USA. 1994;91:2081–5.
32. Ch'ng ES, Jaafar H, Tuan Sharif SE. Breast tumor angiogenesis and tumor-associated macrophages: Histopathologist's perspective. Pathol Res Int. 2011; 13 p. doi:10.4061/2011/572706. Article ID 572706.
33. Reid PE, Brown NJ, Holen I. Breast cancer cells stimulate osteoprotegerin (OPG) production by endothelial cells through direct cell contact. Mol Cancer. 2009;8:49.
34. Cross SS, Yang Z, Brown NJ, et al. Osteoprotegerin (OPG)- a potential new role in the regulation of endothelial cell phenotype and tumour angiogenesis? Int J Cancer. 2006;118(8):1901–8.
35. Hayashida T, Takahashi F, Chiba N, et al. HOXB9, a gene overexpressed in breast cancer, promotes tumorigenicity and lung metastasis. Proc Natl Acad Sci USA. 2010;107(3):1100–5.
36. Greer P. Closing in on the biological functions of Fps/Fes and Fer. Nat Rev Mol Cell Biol. 2002;3(4):278–89.
37. Zhang S, Chitu V, Stanley ER, et al. Fes tyrosine kinase expression in the tumor niche correlates with enhanced tumor growth, angiogenesis, circulating tumor cells, metastasis, and infiltrating macrophages. Cancer Res. 2011;71(4):1465–73.
38. Weidner N, Semple JP, Welch WR, et al. Tumor angiogenesis and metastasis- correlation in invasive breast carcinoma. N Engl J Med. 1991;324(1):1–8.
39. Hansen S, Sørensen FB, Vach W, et al. Microvessel density compared with the Chalkley count in a prognostic study of angiogenesis in breast cancer patients. Histopathology. 2004;44:428–36.
40. McCarthy NJ, Yang X, Linnoila IR, et al. Microvessel density, expression of estrogen receptor alpha, MIB-1, p53, and c-erbB-2 in inflammatory breast cancer. Clin Cancer Res. 2002;8:3857–62.
41. Vermeulen PB, Van Golen KL, Dirix LY. Angiogenesis, lymphangiogenesis, growth pattern, and tumor emboli in inflammatory breast cancer. Cancer. 2010;116 Suppl 11:2748–54.
42. Van der Auwera I, Van Laere SJ, Van den Eynden GG, et al. Increased angiogenesis and lymphangiogenesis in inflammatory versus noninflammatory breast cancer by real-time reverse transcriptase-PCR gene expression quantification. Clin Cancer Res. 2004; 10:7965–71.
43. Bièche I, Lerebours F, Tozlu S, et al. Molecular profiling of inflammatory breast cancer: identification of a poor-prognosis gene expression signature. Clin Cancer Res. 2004;10:6789–95.
44. Shirakawa K, Kobayashi H, Sobajima J, et al. Inflammatory breast cancer. Vasculogenic mimicry and its hemodynamics of an inflammatory breast cancer xenograft model. Breast Cancer Res. 2003; 5:136–9.
45. Mahooti S, Porter K, Alpaugh ML, et al. Breast carcinomatous tumoral emboli can result from encircling lymphovasculogenesis rather than lymphovascular invasion. Oncotarget. 2010;1(2):131–47.
46. Sugino T, Kusakabe T, Hoshi N, et al. An invasion-independent pathway of blood-borne metastasis. A new murine mammary tumor model. Am J Pathol. 2002;160:1973–80.

47. Heimann R, Lan F, McBride R, et al. Separating favorable from unfavorable prognostic markers in breast cancer: the role of E-cadherin. Cancer Res. 2000;60:298–304.
48. Christofori G, Semb H. The role of the cell-adhesion molecule E-cadherin as a tumour-suppressor gene. Trends Biochem Sci. 1999;24:73–6.
49. Alpaugh ML, Tomlinson JS, Shao ZM, et al. A novel human xenograft model of inflammatory breast cancer. Cancer Res. 1999;59:5079–84.
50. Tomlinson JS, Alpaugh ML, Barsky SH. An intact overexpressed E-cadherin/alpha, beta-catenin axis characterizes the lymphovascular emboli of inflammatory breast carcinoma. Cancer Res. 2001;61:5231–41.
51. Hoffmeyer MR, Wall KM, Dharmawardhane SF. *In vitro* analysis of the invasive phenotype of SUM 149, an inflammatory breast cancer cell line. Cancer Cell Int. 2005;5:11.
52. Kleer CG, van Golen KL, Braun T, et al. Persistent E-cadherin expression in inflammatory breast cancer. Mod Pathol. 2001;14:458–64.
53. Colpaert CG, Vermeulen PB, Benoy I, et al. Inflammatory breast cancer shows angiogenesis with high endothelial proliferation rate and strong E-cadherin expression. Br J Cancer. 2003;88:718–25.
54. Liotta LA, Saidel MG, Kleinerman J. The significance of hematogenous tumor cell clumps in the metastatic process. Cancer Res. 1976;36:889–94.
55. Alpaugh ML, Tomlinson JS, Kasraeian S, et al. Cooperative role of E-cadherin and sialyl-Lewis X/A-deficient MUC1 in the passive dissemination of tumor emboli in inflammatory breast carcinoma. Oncogene. 2002;21:3631–43.
56. Alpaugh ML, Barsky SH. Reversible model of spheroid formation allows for high efficiency of gene delivery *ex vivo* and accurate gene assessment *in vivo*. Hum Gene Ther. 2002;13:1245–58.
57. Dong HM, Liu G, Hou YF, et al. Dominant-negative E-cadherin inhibits the invasiveness of inflammatory breast cancer cells *in vitro*. J Cancer Res Clin Oncol. 2007;133:83–92.
58. Silvera D, Arju R, Darvishian F, et al. Essential role for eIF4GI overexpression in the pathogenesis of inflammatory breast cancer. Nat Cell Biol. 2009;11: 903–8.
59. Alpaugh ML, Tomlinson JS, Ye Y, et al. Relationship of sialyl-Lewis(x/a) underexpression and E-cadherin overexpression in the lymphovascular embolus of inflammatory breast carcinoma. Am J Pathol. 2002; 161:619–28.
60. van Golen KL, Wu ZF, Qiao XT, et al. RhoC GTPase, a novel transforming oncogene for human mammary epithelial cells that partially recapitulates the inflammatory breast cancer phenotype. Cancer Res. 2000;60:5832–8.
61. van Golen KL, Davies S, Wu ZF, et al. A novel putative low-affinity insulin-like growth factor-binding protein, LIBC (lost in inflammatory breast cancer), and RhoC-GTPase correlate with the inflammatory breast cancer phenotype. Clin Cancer Res. 1999;5:2511–9.
62. Kleer CG, Zhang Y, Pan Q, et al. *WISP3* is a novel tumor suppressor gene of inflammatory breast cancer. Oncogene. 2002;21:3172–80.
63. Kleer CG, van Golen KL, Zhang Y, et al. Characterization of RhoC expression in benign and malignant breast disease: a potential new marker for small breast carcinomas with metastatic ability. Am J Pathol. 2002;160:579–84.
64. Kleer CG, Griffith KA, Sabel MS, et al. RhoC-GTPase is a novel tissue biomarker associated with biologically aggressive carcinomas of the breast. Breast Cancer Res Treat. 2005;93:101–10.
65. van Golen KL, Wu ZF, Qiao XT, et al. RhoC GTPase overexpression modulates induction of angiogenic factors in breast cells. Neoplasia. 2000;2:418–25.
66. Wu M, Wu ZF, Kumar-Sinha C, et al. RhoC induces differential expression of genes involved in invasion and metastasis in MCF10A breast cells. Breast Cancer Res Treat. 2004;84:3–12.
67. Kleer CG, Zhang Y, Pan Q, et al. WISP3 and RhoC guanosine triphosphatase cooperate in the development of inflammatory breast cancer. Breast Cancer Res. 2004;6:R110–5.
68. Nigro JM, Baker SJ, Preisinger AC, et al. Mutations in the *p53* gene occur in diverse human tumour types. Nature. 1989;342:705–8.
69. Davidoff AM, Humphrey PA, Iglehart JD, et al. Genetic basis for *p53* overexpression in human breast cancer. Proc Natl Acad Sci USA. 1991;88:5006–10.
70. Overmoyer BA. Inflammatory breast cancer: novel preoperative therapies. Clin Breast Cancer. 2010;10:27–32.
71. Moll UM, Riou G, Levine AJ. Two distinct mechanisms alter *p53* in breast cancer: mutation and nuclear exclusion. Proc Natl Acad Sci USA. 1992;89: 7262–6.
72. Riou G, Le MG, Travagli JP, et al. Poor prognosis of *p53* gene mutation and nuclear overexpression of p53 protein in inflammatory breast carcinoma. J Natl Cancer Inst. 1993;85:1765–7.
73. Faille A, De Cremoux P, Extra JM, et al. *p53* mutations and overexpression in locally advanced breast cancers. Br J Cancer. 1994;69:1145–50.
74. Van Laere S, Van der Auwera I, Van den Eynden GG, et al. Distinct molecular signature of inflammatory breast cancer by cDNA microarray analysis. Breast Cancer Res Treat. 2005;93:237–46.
75. Van Laere SJ, Van der Auwera I, Van den Eynden GG, et al. Nuclear factor-kappaB signature of inflammatory breast cancer by cDNA microarray validated by quantitative real-time reverse transcription-PCR, immunohistochemistry, and nuclear factor-kappaB DNA-binding. Clin Cancer Res. 2006;12: 3249–56.
76. Van Laere SJ, Van der Auwera I, Van den Eynden GG, et al. NF-kB activation in inflammatory breast cancer

is associated with oestrogen receptor downregulation, secondary to EGFR and/or ErbB2 overexpression and MAPK hyperactivation. Br J Cancer. 2007;97: 659–69.
77. Cabioglu N, Gong Y, Islam R, et al. Expression of growth factor and chemokine receptors: new insights in the biology of inflammatory breast cancer. Ann Oncol. 2007;18:1021–9.
78. Parrett ML, Harris RE, Joarder FS, Ross MS, Clausen KP, Robertson FM. Cyclooxygenase-2 gene expression in human breast cancer. Int J Oncol. 1997;10:503–7.
79. González-Angulo AM, Guarneri V, Gong Y, et al. Downregulation of the cyclin-dependent kinase inhibitor p27kip1 might correlate with poor disease-free and overall survival in inflammatory breast cancer. Clin Breast Cancer. 2006;7:326–30.
80. Nguyen DM, Sam K, Tsimelzon A, et al. Molecular heterogeneity of inflammatory breast cancer: a hyperproliferative phenotype. Clin Cancer Res. 2006;12: 5047–54.
81. Turpin E, Bièche I, Bertheau P, et al. Increased incidence of ERBB2 overexpression and TP53 mutation in inflammatory breast cancer. Oncogene. 2002;21: 7593–7.
82. Ben Hamida AB, Labidi IS, Mrad K, et al. Markers of subtypes in inflammatory breast cancer studied by immunohistochemistry: prominent expression of P-cadherin. BMC Cancer. 2008;8:28.
83. Charafe-Jauffret E, et al. Immunophenotypic analysis of inflammatory breast cancers: identification of an "inflammatory signature". J Pathol. 2004;202(3):265–73.
84. Van Laere S, Limame R, Van Marck EA, et al. Is there a role for mammary stem cells in inflammatory breast carcinoma? A review of evidence from cell line, animal model, and human tissue sample experiments. Cancer. 2010;116 Suppl 11:2794–805.
85. Smalley M, Ashworth A. Stem cells and breast cancer: a field in transit. Nat Rev Cancer. 2003;3: 832–44.
86. Pardal R, Clarke MF, Morisson SJ. Applying the principles of stem-cell biology to cancer. Nat Rev Cancer. 2003;3:895–902.
87. Diallo R, Schaefer KL, Poremba C, et al. Monoclonality in normal epithelium and in hyperplastic and neoplastic lesions of the breast. J Pathol. 2001;193:27–32.
88. Dontu G, Abdallah WM, Foley JM, et al. *In vitro* propagation and transcriptional profiling of human mammary stem/progenitor cells. Genes Dev. 2003;17:1253–70.
89. Dontu G, Wicha MS. Survival of mammary stem cells in suspension culture: implications for stem cell biology and neoplasia. J Mammary Gland Biol Neoplasia. 2005;10:75–86.
90. Al-Hajj M, Wicha MS, Benito-Hernández A, et al. Prospective identification of tumorigenic breast cancer cells. Proc Natl Acad Sci USA. 2003;100: 3983–8.
91. Ginestier C, Hur MH, Charafe-Jauffret E, et al. ALDH1 is a marker of normal and malignant human mammary stem cells and a predictor of poor clinical outcome. Cell Stem Cell. 2007;1:555–67.
92. Wright MH, Calcagno AM, Salcido CD, et al. Brca1 breast tumors contain distinct CD44þ/CD24- and CD133þ cells with cancer stem cell characteristics. Breast Cancer Res. 2008;10:R10.
93. Smalley MJ, Clarke RB. The mammary gland "side population": a putative stem/progenitor cell marker? J Mammary Gland Biol Neoplasia. 2005;10:37–47.
94. Clayton H, Titley I, Vivanco M. Growth and differentiation of progenitor/stem cells derived from the human mammary gland. Exp Cell Res. 2004;297: 444–60.
95. Bailey JM, Singh PK, Hollingsworth MA. Cancer metastasis facilitated by developmental pathways: sonic hedgehog, notch, and bone morphogenic proteins. J Cell Biochem. 2007;102:829–39.
96. Korkaya H, Paulson A, Charafe-Jauffret E, et al. Regulation of mammary stem/progenitor cells by PTEN/Akt/beta-catenin signaling. PLoS Biol. 2009; 7:e1000121.
97. Xiao Y, Ye Y, Yearsley K, Jones S, Barsky SH. The lymphovascular embolus of inflammatory breast cancer expresses a stem cell-like phenotype. Am J Pathol. 2008;173:561–74.
98. Charafe-Jauffret E, Ginestier C, Iovino F, et al. Breast cancer cell lines contain functional cancer stem cells with metastatic capacity and a distinct molecular signature. Cancer Res. 2009;69:1302–13.
99. Gong Y, González-Angulo AM, Broglio K, et al. Expression of Notch-1 and b-catenin: defining the molecular portrait of inflammatory breast cancer. Breast Cancer Res Treat. 2006;100:S299.
100. Polyak K, Weinberg RA. Transitions between epithelial and mesenchymal states: acquisition of malignant and stem cell traits. Nat Rev Cancer. 2009;9:265–73.
101. Mani SA, Guo W, Liao MJ, et al. The epithelial-mesenchymal transition generates cells with properties of stem cells. Cell. 2008;133:704–15.
102. Zhang D, LaFortune TA, Krishnamurthy S, et al. Epidermal growth factor receptor tyrosine kinase inhibitor reverses mesenchymal to epithelial phenotype and inhibits metastasis in inflammatory breast cancer. Clin Cancer Res. 2009;15:6639–48.
103. Bertucci F, Finetti P, Birnbaum D, et al. Gene expression profiling of inflammatory breast cancer. Cancer. 2010;116 Suppl 11:2783–93.
104. Bertucci F, Finetti P, Rougemont J, et al. Gene expression profiling identifies molecular subtypes of inflammatory breast cancer. Cancer Res. 2005;65: 2170–8.
105. Van Laere SJ, Van den Eynden GG, Van der Auwera I, et al. Identification of cell-of-origin breast tumor subtypes in inflammatory breast cancer by gene expression profiling. Breast Cancer Res Treat. 2006;95:243–55.

106. Van Laere S, Van der Auwera I, Van den Eynden G, et al. Distinct molecular phenotype of inflammatory breast cancer compared to non-inflammatory breast cancer using Affymetrix-based genome-wide gene-expression analysis. Br J Cancer. 2007;97:1165–74.
107. Iwamoto T, Bianchini G, Qi Y, et al. Different gene expressions are associated with the different molecular subtypes of inflammatory breast cancer. Breast Cancer Res Treat. 2011;125:785–95.
108. Boersma BJ, Reimers M, Yi M, et al. A stromal gene signature associated with inflammatory breast cancer. Int J Cancer. 2008;122:1324–32.
109. Van der Auwera I, Limame R, Van Dam P, et al. Integrated miRNA and mRNA expression profiling of the inflammatory breast cancer subtype. Br J Cancer. 2010;103:532–41.

4 Inflammatory Breast Cancer: Clinical Presentation, Diagnosis, Staging Evaluation, Differential Diagnosis, Surgical Treatment, and Follow-Up

Juan Enrique Bargallo-Rocha, Robin J. Shaw-Dulin, Teresa Ramirez-Ugalde, and Angel Herrera-Gomez

Introduction

Inflammatory breast cancer (IBC) is a rare and aggressive form of breast cancer with a relatively poor prognosis. IBC is characterized by the inflammatory appearance of the breast, including diffuse erythema and edema. IBC may be primary, presenting with pain and a tender, firm, and enlarged breast with reddened, warm, and thickened skin. In other cases, IBC may be secondary, characterized by an inflammatory recurrence of a noninflammatory breast cancer, usually developing on the chest wall at the site of a previous mastectomy or rarely as a distant cutaneous recurrence. The signs and symptoms of IBC arise rapidly compared with those that are non-IBC, typically within weeks to 6 months.

A differential diagnosis must be established with noninflammatory locally advanced breast cancer (LABC).

Definition of Inflammatory Breast Cancer

According to the 2010 American Joint Committee on Cancer (AJCC) tumor node metastasis (TNM) breast cancer staging system, inflammatory breast cancer (IBC) is a clinical pathological entity characterized by diffuse erythema and edema (*peau d'orange*) involving one third or more of the skin of the breast [1]. Tumor emboli within the dermal lymph nodes are responsible for these skin changes, which are classified as primary tumor stage T4d and which are staged as either IIIB, IIIC, or IV.

The Gustave-Roussy classification uses the poussee evolutive (PEV) breast cancer classification based on rate of development and extent of involvement of the breast and recognizes the following: PEV 0 as a tumor with no recent increase in size or presence of inflammatory signs; PEV 1 as a tumor with an increase in size over the last 2 months with no inflammatory signs; PEV 2 as a tumor with inflammatory signs of edema, erythema, and warmth involving less than one half of the breast skin surface; and PEV 3 as a tumor with inflammatory signs involving more than one half of the breast skin surface. In accordance with this system, IBC is PEV 2 or PEV 3.

J.E. Bargallo-Rocha, M.D. (✉)
Department of Breast Cancer,
Instituto Nacional de Cancerologia-Mexico,
Avenida San Fernando 22, Tlalpan, Mexico City,
DF 014804, Mexico
e-mail: ebargallo@incan.edu.mx

R.J. Shaw-Dulin, M.D. • T. Ramirez-Ugalde, M.D.
Department of Breast Tumors,
Instituto Nacional de Cancerologia-Mexico,
Mexico City, DF, Mexico

A. Herrera-Gomez, M.D.
Department of Surgical Oncology,
Instituto Nacional de Cancerologia-Mexico,
Mexico City, DF, Mexico

J.G. de la Garza-Salazar et al. (eds.), *Inflammatory Breast Cancer*,
DOI 10.1007/978-0-85729-991-8_4, © Springer-Verlag London 2013

At the National Institute of Cancer in Mexico (INCan), we employ the AJCC TNM classification system.

Diagnosis of IBC is based on the clinical presentation. Although dermal lymph node involvement supports the diagnosis, it is neither necessary nor sufficient in the absence of classical clinical findings.

Clinical Presentation

Patients with IBC typically present with pain and a rapidly progressing, tender, firm, and enlarged breast. The skin of the breast is warm and thickened, with a *peau d'orange* (orange skin) appearance. Skin color can range from an initial pink-flushed discoloration to redness or to a purplish hue that appears to represent ecchymosis. At presentation, nearly all women with IBC have lymph node involvement, and approximately one third have distant metastases [2–4].

There is increasing epidemiologic and molecular evidence suggesting that IBC represents a distinct disease entity rather than forming part of the spectrum of LABC, making accurate differentiation crucial to ensure proper treatment. In the absence of a specific histopathological subtype and due to debate regarding the relevance of dermal lymph node invasion, IBC is universally recognized as a clinical diagnosis [5–7].

Historically, the first description of the disease was attributed to Sir Charles Bell, who in 1814 described "a purple color on the skin over the tumor accompanied by shooting pains." In 1924, Lee and Tannenbaum coined the term "inflammatory breast cancer" when describing the features of a 28-patient series. Their classic description follows here: "As the disease progresses, the skin becomes deep red or reddish-purple, and to the touch is brawny and infiltrated. The inflamed area presents a distinct raised periphery after the fashion of erysipelas. The examiner with his eyes closed… can distinguish the sharp contrast between normal and affected tissue."

In 1938, Taylor and Meltzer first assigned the terms "primary IBC" or "true IBC" and "secondary IBC" when describing two clinical varieties of the inflammatory changes of breast cancer. Primary IBC was utilized to describe the simultaneous development of inflammatory skin changes and carcinoma in a previously normal breast. Secondary IBC described inflammatory changes in a breast that already had cancer or following a mastectomy for noninflammatory breast cancer.

In light of the wide spectrum of clinical presentations included in the application of the term IBC, Haagensen established specific diagnostic criteria to describe true IBC in 1956, including rapid enlargement of the breast, generalized induration in the presence or absence of a distinct breast palpable mass, edema of the skin of the breast, erythema that must involve more than one third of the breast, and biopsy-proven carcinoma. These criteria continue to be used for diagnosis today. Flattening, crusting, and nipple retraction can also occur as the disease progress.

Clinical Signs and Symptoms

Patients with IBC often present with symptoms such as a sensation of heaviness, aching, or burning of the breast, leading to clinical signs within a short time interval due to the rapid progression that characterizes this entity. Either breast may be affected, yet some series have described a predilection for the left breast. IBC more frequently affects females, as with all breast cancer. Patients tend to be younger at diagnosis (58 vs. 61 years of age) and are more likely to be pre- or perimenopausal.

The first clinical sign of IBC comprises skin changes that vary in color and distribution patterns depending on the extent of disease at presentation. In early stage disease, erythema ranges from light pink to mottled pink in color. The discoloration tends to be more prominent in the lower, dependent half of the breast. As the disease advances, erythema intensifies to a dark red or purple color that spreads diffusely to encompass the whole breast. As these skin changes are often nonspecific, IBC is frequently misdiagnosed as a benign inflammatory process, leading to significant delays due to the use of antibiotics and drainage attempts of the presumed breast abscess. Because true inflammation is not present in IBC, systemic symptoms and signs suggesting a true inflammatory process, such as fever and leukocytosis, should not be present.

Other causes for delayed diagnosis include difficulty in identifying skin changes in darker skin, which may account for the higher proportion of advanced disease at presentation and poorer prognosis in African-American women.

As erythema may involve the overlying skin of the breast in locally advanced breast cancer, erythematous changes must involve one third of the breast in order to qualify as IBC.

Rapid enlargement of the breast is pathognomonic of IBC, occurring nearly simultaneously with skin changes. The involved breast may double or triple its original size within a few weeks.

The rapid rate of disease progression (usually within a 10-week interval) with associated erythema affecting more than one third of the skin overlying the breast distinguishes true IBC from a neglected locally advanced cancer that has developed inflammatory changes over time.

The frequent absence of an underlying breast mass should increase suspicion of IBC. Specific skin manifestations associated with IBC also include *peau d'orange* or orange skin, first described by Leitch in 1909 when observing the appearance of exaggerated hair follicle pits associated with skin edema. *Peau d'orange* may compromise the entire breast, yet it is usually more evident in the dependent part of the breast.

Ulceration does not generally occur in IBC and is more indicative of neglected LABC.

Fixed palpable ipsilateral axillary lymph nodes are a frequent finding (up to 100 % of patients upon diagnosis in some series), in addition to the involvement of supraclavicular nodes. Extreme cases of nodal involvement may lead to arm lymphedema.

Up to one third of patients will have distant metastases at diagnosis. Disease progression involving the opposite breast and contralateral axillary lymph nodes can occur. Bilateral synchronous breast involvement may also take place [17].

Differential Diagnosis

Several conditions may be confused with IBC, leading to delays in diagnosis and treatment:[30].

- Infectious mastitis and breast abscess: Early stage IBC may often mimic benign inflammatory processes. These conditions typically occur in lactating women and are generally associated with localized tenderness, fever, and leukocytosis. To avoid misdiagnosis, patients with skin changes of the breast persisting for >10–14 days despite treatment with antibiotics should be referred for further investigation, including breast biopsy:
  - Lactational mastitis: The most common form of infectious mastitis.
  - Breast abscess: The majority of breast abscesses are a complication of mastitis.
  - Tuberculous mastitis — Tuberculosis (TB) of the breast is rare. Clinical presentation is usually a solitary, ill-defined, unilateral hard lump. TB can also present with nipple discharge, skin thickening, or discharging sinuses in the breast or axillae [31].

  Breast TB can mimic breast carcinoma or breast abscess both clinically and radiologically. Mammographic imaging may show a dense tract connecting an ill-defined breast mass to an area of skin thickening and a skin bulge. Ultrasound (US) may demonstrate a complex, predominantly cystic mass. Solid caseating granulomata may be observed on biopsy. Diagnosis of TB is made by identification of acid-fast bacillus or by positive cultures.

  The disease is curable with antitubercular drugs, and surgery is rarely required. Treatment should follow standard recommendations for systemic tuberculosis.
  - Other infectious causes of mastitis: Primary actinomycosis, syphilis, and mycotic, helminthic, and viral infections have all been reported in the breast.
- Noninfectious mastitis: Includes entities such as periductal mastitis and idiopathic granulomatous mastitis. These entities do not necessarily occur during lactation, they are not

always accompanied by a microbial infection, and they may not resolve with antibiotic therapy:

– *Idiopathic granulomatous mastitis*: Idiopathic granulomatous mastitis (IGM, also known as idiopathic granulomatous lobular mastitis) is a rare benign inflammatory disease of the breast of unknown etiology. IGM is most commonly observed in parous young women, often within a few years of pregnancy. There is no increased risk of subsequent breast cancer in patients with IGM.

  IGM is most frequently diagnosed following the development of a peripheral inflammatory mass, which may be confused with cancer on physical examination and imaging studies. IGM can also present as a single hard breast mass or as multiple simultaneous areas of peripheral infection with abscesses and/or overlying skin inflammation and ulceration. Nipple retraction, sinus formation, *peau d'orange*-like changes, and axillary adenopathy may accompany the preceding findings. Women with IGM may develop repeated abscesses over durations ranging from weeks to months.

  Patients with IGM may have symptoms and signs that may be mistaken for nonpuerperal mastitis, a breast abscess, or carcinoma. The mammographic findings of IGM, like the physical findings, are often suggestive of malignancy. US examination in such instances typically shows a solid mass, often with abscesses.

  IGM is a diagnosis of exclusion, as there are several processes such as sarcoidosis or tuberculosis of the breast that may also induce granulomatous mastitis. A core needle biopsy of a solid mass should be performed to confirm the diagnosis of IGM. Biopsy findings typically show granulomatous lesions that are centered on the breast lobule. When IGM is suspected, the biopsy specimen should be sent for acid-fast bacillus and fungal stains in addition to histopathology.

  Treatment: IGM associated with localized infection will usually resolve with antibiotics and drainage.

  Although systemic glucocorticoid therapy has been used successfully to treat symptomatic patients, based on the hypothesis that this is an autoimmune disease, there are no randomized controlled trials that demonstrate efficacy for glucocorticoids in the treatment of IGM. It is not clear whether steroids influence the course of this condition, which often resolves spontaneously if left untreated. Thus, many have abandoned steroids for treatment of IGM. Methotrexate has also been employed successfully for treatment of IGM in several case reports. However, steroids and methotrexate both have adverse side effects, and symptoms frequently rebound with increased inflammation when these drugs are discontinued.

  Surgical excision or mastectomy for IGM is often followed by prolonged wound healing and is not recommended.

- Radiation dermatitis: Skin changes in the conserved breast resembling IBC can occur following radiation therapy. These skin changes are usually sharply delimited, confined to the radiation port, and take place after the second or third week of therapy. These skin changes frequently fade after 2–3 weeks, leaving pigmented skin behind after desquamation of the skin occurs.
- Lymphoma or leukemia — Involvement of the breast by these malignant breast lesions may be clinically indistinguishable from IBC [28, 29].

Primary lymphoma of the breast is extremely rare, accounting for 0.04–0.5 % of all breast malignancies and approximately 1–2 % of all extranodal lymphomas. On the other hand, secondary involvement of the breast with lymphomas is not uncommon.

The majority of breast lymphoma present as a unilateral painless breast mass in an older woman (average age at diagnosis, 55–60 years). For unknown reasons, the right breast is involved more often than the left. Ipsilateral axillary lymphadenopathy is present in 30–40 % of cases. There is some evidence that widespread mammographic screening for breast carcinoma is leading to increased incidental detection of lymphoma of the breast.

A less common but distinctive presentation comprises that of a young woman of childbearing age who presents during or immediately after pregnancy. The disease is often bilateral and may clinically mimic inflammatory breast cancer. The majority of these women have highly aggressive Burkitt's lymphoma.

Systemic "B" symptoms (fever, weight loss, night sweats) are uncommon.

Published clinical and histological criteria for a diagnosis of primary (as opposed to secondary) breast lymphoma include the following:

- A pathological specimen with close association between the lymphomatous infiltrate and the breast tissue.
- No evidence of widespread disease or prior extramammary lymphoma.
- The breast is the principal site of involvement, but ipsilateral axillary lymph node involvement is acceptable if both lesions develop simultaneously.

Although a core biopsy is adequate for performing a diagnosis of breast lymphoma, excisional biopsy is preferable. Radiographically, breast lymphomas appear as nonspecific circumscribed masses that lack calcification or evidence of a desmoplastic reaction (i.e., retraction), but these features are nonspecific.

As with other lymphomas, primary breast lymphomas are staged according to the Ann Arbor Staging System. In general, treatment of primary breast lymphomas follows treatment recommendations for lymphomas of the same stage and histology at other locations. Choice of chemotherapy regimen should be based on histological subtype, disease extent, and the individual patient:

- Noninflammatory locally advanced breast cancer or a breast cancer recurrence involving the skin that causes late inflammation is sometimes difficult to differentiate from true IBC.
- Congestive heart failure: Rare causes of unilateral breast swelling have been described with congestive heart failure, although bilateral breast edema is more common. These patients present with physical signs and nonspecific mammographic findings consistent with IBC. Some describe pitting edema of the breast as a method for differentiating heart failure from IBC.

Diagnosis and Staging Evaluation

There are no specific laboratory markers that correlate with the diagnosis of IBC and mammographic imaging is often not specific. Clinical features may be suggestive of IBC; however, biopsy for histological confirmation is essential [17]. Specimens for pathological study may be obtained by core needle biopsy guided by palpation, sonography, or stereotactic radiography. A full-thickness skin biopsy is often obtained if IBC is suspected because a hallmark of this disease is dermal lymphatic invasion by tumor cells.

IBC is always classified as T4d and is assigned at least a stage IIIB according to AJCC TNM staging criteria.

As with LABC, palpable or suspicious lymph nodes may be evaluated with US of the axillae with guided fine-needle aspiration (FNA) and/or a core needle biopsy in order to arrive at a more accurate determination of the tumor stage.

Once the diagnosis has been confirmed, an appropriate initial workup should include additional laboratory and imaging studies to evaluate for bone, liver, or pulmonary metastases, given the increased risk of distant metastases.

Staging evaluation should include the following:

- Clinical history and physical examination
- Diagnostic bilateral mammography and breast US
- Laboratory tests, including a complete blood count with platelets, liver function tests, alkaline phosphatase
- Imaging studies including chest X-ray or chest computed tomography (CT), abdominal US or abdominal CT, bone scan, positron emission tomography (PET) CT
- Histological confirmation of malignancy
- *Very* important currently in the management of advanced noninflammatory breast cancer (nIBC) (T4) are the following studies:
  - Hormonal receptors (ER/PR), BRC 1 and 2, EGFR (HER2/c-neu), p 52, and cadherin-E

Clinical history will document a rapid onset of the disease process usually within a few weeks to 6 months.

Physical examination will reveal the characteristic skin features discussed previously (erythema affecting at least one third of the breast, thickening or fine dimpling, edema, warmth, and a palpable ridge at the margin of induration), a distinct palpable mass in only 50 % of patients, and the presence of palpable or matted axillary lymph nodes because nearly all women with IBC have nodal involvement.

Mammography may show an obvious tumor mass, large areas of calcification, or parenchymal distortion in 80–90 % of patients, while 10–15 % of these present only with mammographic signs of inflammation, such as characteristic skin thickening over the breast, stromal coarsening, increased vascularity, or diffuse opacity. Bilateral mammography is essential for the diagnosis of occult lesions in the same or in the contralateral breast.

Ultrasonography is very helpful in the evaluation of regional nodal status, with positive axillary nodes in >90 % of patients with IBC. The proportion of patients with metastasis in infraclavicular, supraclavicular, and internal mammary nodes is approximately 50, 33, and 13 %, respectively.

There is limited data on the value of additional imaging studies of the breast, including magnetic resonance imaging (MRI), CT, or PET, in the diagnostic evaluation of IBC [8, 9].

Radiological examinations aimed at detecting the presence of distant metastatic disease should be performed as indicated by the patient's history or physical examination findings. In the asymptomatic patient, these studies should include bone scan; chest, abdominal, and head CT; and liver function and alkaline phosphatase tests to guide detection of liver or bone metastasis. At diagnosis, approximately 25 % of patients with IBC will have distant metastasis.

Treatment

Any breast cancer (including LABC and IBC) can be detected by mammography, but some cases are easily palpable (some with a long time prior to diagnosis). Previous studies plus needle aspiration provide information on tumor grade and ER, PR, and HER2/neu status. p53 and Ki67 may also be utilized to confirm lymph node metastasis.

Locoregional Treatment of Inflammatory Breast Cancer

Inflammatory breast cancer (IBC) is an aggressive form of locally advanced breast cancer (LABC). Multimodality therapy with neoadjuvant chemotherapy followed by locoregional therapy has become the standard approach [25]. While anthracycline- and taxane-containing regimens are most commonly recommended, the optimal chemotherapy regimen and sequencing of agents have yet to be defined [27].

Historically, single modality therapy for IBC was undertaken on the basis of the presumption that the best chance for a cure was found with the most radical operation possible: the Halsted radical mastectomy. Halsted's original experience printed in 1894 in the JH Hospital Bulletin was reported in patients with LABC, none of these fitting modern descriptions of IBC. Later series such as those by Haagensen [35] reported 30 patients treated by radical mastectomy with a mean survival of 19 months. Treves reported a series of 114 patients—the largest at the time—with only 3.5 % of patients alive after 5 years of being treated with radical mastectomy [26]. (Treves, Surg Gynecol Obstet 1959). This led authors to conclude that radical mastectomy was contraindicated in the treatment of patients with IBC because the disease was usually disseminated at the time of diagnosis. Haagensen and Stout in 1942 defined the concepts of operable and inoperable breast cancer, still employed today, and radiotherapy, which to that point had been utilized for patients who were not candidates for mastectomy, became the primary treatment modality.

Local control rates and mean survival remained poor using single modality therapy, with 5-year overall survival rates of <10 % for mastectomy alone or for definitive radiation therapy (RT).

Authors in the 1970s proposed combining surgery and RT for improved locoregional control, but this exerted no impact on survival [10]. With the adoption of neoadjuvant chemotherapy, outcomes for IBC have improved as follows:

- Series of patients treated with neoadjuvant chemotherapy followed by surgery and RT have reported 5-year disease-free survival (DFS) rates of 20–45 % and overall survival (OS) rates of 30–70 % [8, 10–15].
- Patients who obtain a complete pathologic response from chemotherapy have significantly higher disease-free survival and overall survival [10–12, 14–16].
- The combined local approach of surgery and RT following neoadjuvant chemotherapy provides optimal locoregional control but appears to have no impact on OS [10].

Modern Concepts in Surgical Treatment for IBC

In general, women with IBC are approached similarly to those with noninflammatory LABC with a multidisciplinary team (Radiologist, Pathologist, Medical Oncologist, Surgeons, and Radiation Oncologists). Breast conservation therapy is generally considered inappropriate for these women. [32–34]

Following neoadjuvant chemotherapy, standard locoregional treatment includes mastectomy and RT. Patients who do not achieve optimal tumor debulking or who remain inoperable should receive RT with subsequent surgery, if possible.

In general, locoregional management decisions are based on tumor response. Patients who achieve a pathologic complete remission compared to those with a lesser response have significantly higher DFS and OS, whereas patients with extensive residual disease after NCT have a poor prognosis [10, 11, 14–16, 18]. The combined local approach of surgery and RT following neoadjuvant chemotherapy provides optimal locoregional control but may only minimally impact OS [10]. Surgery generally precedes RT because higher RT doses can be more safely delivered in the post- compared with the preoperative setting [13, 19].

Surgery

The goals of surgery in IBC are to maintain local control and to improve survival. Mastectomy as primary treatment has long been recognized as insufficient, with several case series reported between 1920 and 1950 providing evidence of poor survival and local control. The poor outcome of surgical treatment resulted in RT becoming the primary therapeutic treatment modality for the management of IBC until the 1970s.

Studies focusing on neoadjuvant chemotherapy administration in the 1970s suggested a prolongation of disease-free survival and OS compared with historical controls, introducing the necessity for multimodality therapy and local control.

Mastectomy is generally considered an integral part of the multimodality treatment of IBC, although some have questioned whether mastectomy can be replaced with breast conservation surgery or RT alone, especially for patients who achieve a complete clinical response to neoadjuvant chemotherapy [20–22]. However, others have shown in case series that mastectomy improves local control, DFS, and cancer-specific survival [10, 23].

In the absence of definitive data produced by prospective randomized trials, the theoretical advantages to mastectomy include the following:

1. Histological examination of the mastectomy specimen allows a more accurate evaluation of response than clinical or imaging evaluation. The degree of pathological response is an important indicator of prognosis after neoadjuvant therapy. Findings from the mastectomy specimen may influence decisions concerning the need for additional systemic therapy.
2. Mastectomy has the potential of removing foci of chemoresistant disease, potentially improving local control.

Postmastectomy chest wall RT is generally recommended for patients with LABC and IBC who are treated with neoadjuvant chemotherapy followed by mastectomy. Although a survival benefit for postmastectomy RT has not been definitively proven in patients with IBC, the improvement in locoregional control renders RT an important part of the management of these patients.

Selection Criteria for Surgical Treatment in Patients with IBC

Patients who present clinical evidence of IBC should be considered inoperable at presentation.

Surgery should only be attempted if a macroscopically complete resection can be accomplished [24]. Patients are considered candidates for modified radical mastectomy when all evidence of skin inflammation has resolved in response to chemotherapy; surgery in patients who do not respond to chemotherapy is associated with both poor survival and poor local control. There have been reports of chest wall recurrence as early as the second postoperative week when surgery is performed without resolution of inflammatory skin changes. Therefore, chemotherapy should be followed by radiotherapy when skin inflammation persists. Standard criteria for inoperability also apply in IBC: supraclavicular adenopathy, fixed axillary lymphadenopathy, and edema of the ipsilateral arm all comprise an indication for RT for local control.

Sentinel Lymph Node Biopsy in Patients with IBC

Although sentinel lymph node biopsy is increasingly accepted as a valid procedure to predict axillary nodal status in patients after neoadjuvant chemotherapy, IBC has long been considered a contraindication. It is thought that lymphatics may be blocked with tumor cells, rendering the migration of blue dye and/or radiocolloid to regional lymph nodes impossible. Published reports on sentinel lymph node biopsy after neoadjuvant chemotherapy in patients with IBC have reported high rates of failure in identifying a sentinel lymph node and false-negative results [34].

Breast Reconstruction in Patients with IBC

The role of immediate breast reconstruction in locally advanced disease is controversial. Concerns include delays in the administration of postoperative therapies if problems with wound healing occur, the negative effect of RT on the cosmetic outcome of the reconstruction, and the high risks of local recurrence.

There are very few published series on the use of immediate breast reconstruction in patients with IBC because the development of local recurrence is frequent. Moreover, skin-sparing mastectomy should be avoided due to the inability to ensuring eradication of all malignant cells in the skin with preoperative chemotherapy and the negative cosmetic effects of routine postoperative radiation.

Delayed reconstruction should be chosen over immediate reconstruction in patients who have completed oncologic therapy.

Follow-Up

The goals of posttreatment surveillance after primary treatment for breast cancer are early recognition and treatment of disease recurrences, second primary breast cancers, and therapy-related complications.

References

1. Edge SB, Byrd DR, Compton CC, et al., editors. AJCC (American Joint Committee on Cancer) cancer staging manual. 7th ed. New York: Springer; 2010.
2. Hance KW, Anderson WF, Devesa SS, et al. Trends in inflammatory breast carcinoma incidence and survival: the surveillance, epidemiology, and end results program at the National Cancer Institute. J Natl Cancer Inst. 2005;97:966.
3. Anderson WF, Schairer C, Chen BE, et al. Epidemiology of inflammatory breast cancer (IBC). Breast Dis. 2005–2006;22:9.
4. Tai P, Yu E, Shiels R, et al. Short- and long-term cause-specific survival of patients with inflammatory breast cancer. BMC Cancer. 2005;5:137.
5. Kleer CG, van Golen KL, Merajver SD. Molecular biology of breast cancer metastasis. Inflammatory breast cancer: clinical syndrome and molecular determinants. Breast Cancer Res. 2000;2:423.
6. Jaiyesimi IA, Buzdar AU, Hortobagyi G. Inflammatory breast cancer: a review. J Clin Oncol. 1992;10:1014.
7. Walshe JM, Swain SM. Clinical aspects of inflammatory breast cancer. Breast Dis. 2005–2006;22:35.
8. Smoot RL, Koch CA, Degnim AC, et al. A single-center experience with inflammatory breast cancer, 1985–2003. Arch Surg. 2006;141:567.

9. Chow CK. Imaging in inflammatory breast carcinoma. Breast Dis. 2005–2006;22:45.
10. Pérez CA, Fields JN, Fracasso PM, et al. Management of locally advanced carcinoma of the breast. II. Inflammatory carcinoma. Cancer. 1994;74:466.
11. Thoms Jr WW, McNeese MD, Fletcher GH, et al. Multimodal treatment for inflammatory breast cancer. Int J Radiat Oncol Biol Phys. 1989;17:739.
12. Baldini E, Gardin G, Evagelista G, et al. Long-term results of combined-modality therapy for inflammatory breast carcinoma. Clin Breast Cancer. 2004;5:358.
13. Liauw SL, Benda RK, Morris CG, Mendenhall NP. Inflammatory breast carcinoma: outcomes with trimodality therapy for nonmetastatic disease. Cancer. 2004;100:920.
14. Harris EE, Schultz D, Bertsch H, et al. Ten-year outcome after combined modality therapy for inflammatory breast cancer. Int J Radiat Oncol Biol Phys. 2003;55:1200.
15. Palangie T, Mosseri V, Mihura J, et al. Prognostic factors in inflammatory breast cancer and therapeutic implications. Eur J Cancer. 1994;30A:921.
16. Hennessy BT, González-Angulo AM, Hortobagyi GN, et al. Disease-free and overall survival after pathologic complete disease remission of cytologically proven inflammatory breast carcinoma axillary lymph node metastases after primary systemic chemotherapy. Cancer. 2006;106:1000.
17. Harris J., Lippman M., Morrow M., Osborne C. Diseases of the Breast 4th Edition. 2009.
18. Cristofanilli M, Buzdar AU, Hortobágyi GN. Update on the management of inflammatory breast cancer. Oncologist. 2003;8:141.
19. Liao Z, Strom EA, Buzdar AU, et al. Locoregional irradiation for inflammatory breast cancer: effectiveness of dose escalation in decreasing recurrence. Int J Radiat Oncol Biol Phys. 2000;47:1191.
20. De Boer RH, Allum WH, Ebbs SR, et al. Multimodality therapy in inflammatory breast cancer: is there a place for surgery? Ann Oncol. 2000;11:1147.
21. Brun B, Otmezguine Y, Feuilhade F, et al. Treatment of inflammatory breast cancer with combination chemotherapy and mastectomy versus breast conservation. Cancer. 1988;61:1096.
22. Bristol IJ, Buchholz TA. Inflammatory breast cancer: current concepts in local management. Breast Dis. 2005–2006;22:75.
23. Panades M, Olivotto IA, Speers CH, et al. Evolving treatment strategies for inflammatory breast cancer: a population-based survival analysis. J Clin Oncol. 2005;23:1941.
24. Curcio LD, Rupp E, Williams WL, et al. Beyond palliative mastectomy in inflammatory breast cancer – a reassessment of margin status. Ann Surg Oncol. 1999;6:249.
25. Pisansky TM, Schaid DJ, Loprinzi CL, et al. Inflammatory breast cancer: integration of irradiation, surgery, and chemotherapy. Am J Clin Oncol. 1992; 15:376.
26. TREVES N. The inoperability of inflammatory carcinoma of the breast. Surg Gynecol Obstet. 1959 Aug; 109 (2):240–242.
27. Cristofanilli M, Valero V, Buzdar AU, et al. Inflammatory breast cancer (IBC) and patterns of recurrence: understanding the biology of a unique disease. Cancer. 2007;110:1436.
28. Talwalkar SS, Miranda RN, Valbuena JR, et al. Lymphomas involving the breast: a study of 106 cases comparing localized and disseminated neoplasms. Am J Surg Pathol. 2008;32:1299.
29. Wong WW, Schild SE, Halyard MY, Schomberg PJ. Primary non-Hodgkin lymphoma of the breast: the mayo clinic experience. J Surg Oncol. 2002;80:19.
30. Kamal RM, Hamed ST, Salem DS. Classification of inflammatory breast disorders and step by step diagnosis. Breast J. 2009;15:367.
31. Baharoon S. Tuberculosis of the breast. Ann Thorac Med. 2008;3:110.
32. De la Garza-Salazar, JG, et al. Different management of inflammatory breast cancer. In: American Society of clinical oncology (meeting), Abstract C-32, Denver, 1977.
33. De la Garza J, et al. Cancer inflamatorio de la glándula mamaria. Experiencia de 6 años con Qt. Rt. Cir Ciruj (Mexico) 1977;45(6):351–7.
34. Kell MR, Marrow M. Surgical aspects of inflammatory breast cancer. Breast Dis. 2005–2006;22:67–73.
35. Haagensen CD (1971) Diseases of the Breast 2nd edn, Philadelphia: WB Saunders Company.

Imaging in Inflammatory Carcinoma

5

Yolanda Villaseñor-Navarro, Lesvia Olivia Aguilar-Cortazar, Irma Perez-Zuñiga, Roberto Alejandro Cruz-Morales, Cecilia Magdalena Pavon-Hernandez, Martha Patricia Perez-Badillo, and Jaime Ignacio Garcia-Gomez

Inflammatory carcinoma (IC) is a rare and aggressive form of primary epithelial cancer that constitutes 1–6 % of breast cancer. It is found associated with poor prognosis, given the high probability of micrometastasis at the time of diagnosis; likewise, about 20 % of patients have distant metastasis on diagnosis [1], with a high incidence of recurrence, greater than that of noninflammatory cancers.

Inflammatory breast cancer is clinically diagnosed by the rapid appearance of erythema and edema denominated by "orange skin" (*peau d'orange*) that involves at least one third of the skin that surrounds the mammary gland.

The primary tumor of IC is classified as T4d by definition, even when an apparent mass is not identified in the breast. When inflammatory breast cancer is manifested, the majority of women present lymph node involvement, and approximately one third of these women have distant disease.

Despite the term "inflammatory," the clinical characteristics are due to blockage of dermal lymphatic emboli-associated drainage of the skin. Differential diagnosis of this pathology includes mastitis and cellulitis of the breast [2–4].

The classical criteria for the clinical diagnosis of inflammatory breast carcinoma (IBC) were established by Haagensen in 1971 [5]: increase in volume and pain, swelling and heat, *peau d'orange*, inverted nipple, and inflamed breast. Symptoms progress rapidly, and the majority of patients tend to have axillary lymph node commitment on IBC presentation.

The breast is typically increased in volume, hot, and painful to the touch; flatness and nipple retraction are frequently observed, especially as the disease progresses. There is consensus at present concerning that the diagnosis of IBC is clinically eminent.

No laboratory abnormality has been associated with IBC, and in general, there is the presence of neither leukocytosis nor fever.

However, an initial biopsy is preferred for diagnosis, obtaining adequate samples of the tumor, the skin, and the skin lymph nodes.

The lack of specificity of some symptoms and the lack of suspicion of this entity cause many women with IBC to be poorly diagnosed, confusing the former with symptoms of mastitis, these being the main causes of delay in diagnosis and treatment of the disease.

Infectious mastitis and abscesses tend to occur in lactating women, with associated fever and leukocytosis, which occur with little frequency in IBC. Lymphosarcomatous involvement and leukemia of the breast can be difficult to distinguish clinically and require histologic or cytologic

Y. Villaseñor-Navarro (✉) • L.O. Aguilar-Cortazar
I. Perez-Zuñiga • R.A. Cruz-Morales
C.M. Pavon-Hernandez • M.P. Perez-Badillo
J.I. Garcia-Gomez
Department of Radiology, Instituto Nacional de Cancerologia-Mexico,
Avenida San Fernando 22, Tlalpan,
Mexico City, DF 14080, Mexico
e-mail: yolavillana@hotmail.com

J.G. de la Garza-Salazar et al. (eds.), *Inflammatory Breast Cancer*,
DOI 10.1007/978-0-85729-991-8_5, © Springer-Verlag London 2013

examination in order to afford an exact diagnosis; less frequently, other diseases, such as syphilis and tuberculosis, can produce inflammatory changes in the breast [6] (Fig. 5.1a, b).

Differentiation between benign inflammatory pathology and inflammatory cancer (IC) represents a challenge due to the similar characteristics between these two conditions.

On the other hand, even the definition of IBC differs. According to multiple studies reported, IBC is frequently included within the classification of locally advanced carcinoma with secondary inflammatory changes, which generally presents a large mass and changes in the skin as well as its evolution [7, 8]. Buzdar et al. [9] suggest the presence of two different clinical entities: on the one hand, primary IBC of the breast and, on the other, locally advanced breast carcinoma (LABC) with secondary inflammatory changes, each with different tendencies with respect to incidence and survival curves.

The importance of imaging studies in the evaluation of IBC not only defines evaluation of the primary lesion but also is important in delimitation of the extension, follow-up, etc. [10]:

1. Characterization of primary tumor to facilitate guided imaging biopsy
2. Delimiting locoregional disease
3. Diagnosis of distant metastasis
4. Evaluation of treatment response

During the last decade, there have been dramatic advances in the imaging techniques employed for the detection and diagnosis of breast cancer, including IBC: conventional or analog mammography, digital ultrasound (US) mammography, magnetic resonance (MR), positron emission tomography-computed tomography (PET-CT), and positron emission mammography (PET), which have improved the diagnosis and staging of the disease.

IC has mammographic patterns of inflammatory changes, considering among these thickening of the skin, trabecular thickening, and diffuse increase of parenchyma density, findings that are manifested on comparison with the contralateral breast. Other findings present are distortion, nipple retraction, and the possible presence of a primary tumor and/or microcalcifications [11] (Fig. 5.2a, b).

Trabecular and diffuse skin thickening are the most frequent alterations of IC, but these are not specific because they also tend to be associated with mastitis (Fig. 5.1) and locally advanced cancer with inflammatory changes, which usually manifest as a large-sized mass with localized skin changes adjacent to this mass [12].

Cutaneous thickness should not exceed 2.5–3 mm, and mammographically, this finding first manifests in the subareolar region and later extends to the entire breast. This finding aids in differentiating IC from other inflammatory processes that exhibit focal or segmentary cutaneous thickening.

Mammary tissue can show signs of inflammation after surgery or radiotherapy (RT) and in different benign disorders such as trauma, infection, and dermatosis. Superior vena cava thrombosis or congestive heart and lymphatic failure have also been reported as extramammary causes of breast edema [13] (Fig. 5.3a, b).

It is important to consider mammary parenchyma density according to the mammographic parameters described by the American College of Radiology (ACR) [14] because this contributes to the low and high density of the primary lesions in the mammography, as well as of multifocality or multicentricity and even bilaterality [1]. It is estimated that average age at presentation of IC is 51 years and that >90 % of patients will have dense breasts, which leads to poor visualization of the mammographic characteristics of IC, including nodules, microcalcifications, and skin changes [13]. One limiting factor is the possible difficulty of performing an optimal mammography in patients with important inflammation and pain that does not permit compression.

Digital mammography in the diagnosis of IC is as limited as conventional mammography, mainly due to high mammary density; despite this, the former has allowed for better assessment of skin thickening, trabecular alterations, and increased stromal density. With the advent of increased advanced applications, such as tomosynthesis and the application of contrast medium

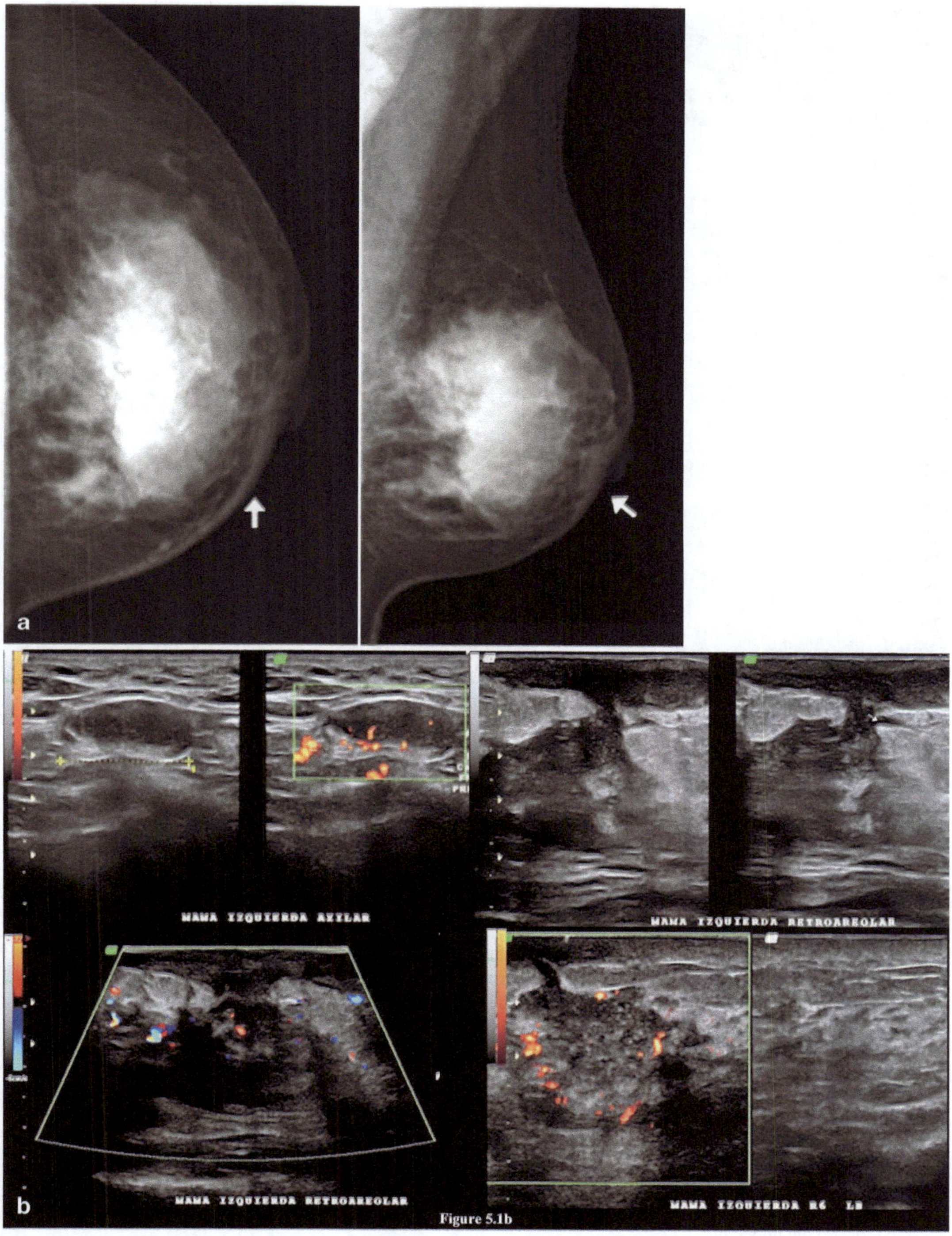

Fig. 5.1 (**a**) Left mammography in caudal cranial projections and mediolateral oblique mean. Identification of thickening of the periareolar skin and in inferior internal quadrants (*arrows*), likewise an increase in breast parenchyma density toward the interline of the quadrants associated with distortion of mammary architecture. (**b**) Ultrasound shows skin thickening and the presence of heterogeneous hypoechoic images, irregular, with vascularity on application of Doppler color that fistulize toward the skin. Axillary lymph nodes with cortical thickening. Antibiotic therapy was administered, resolving the clinical picture 3 weeks after its initiation

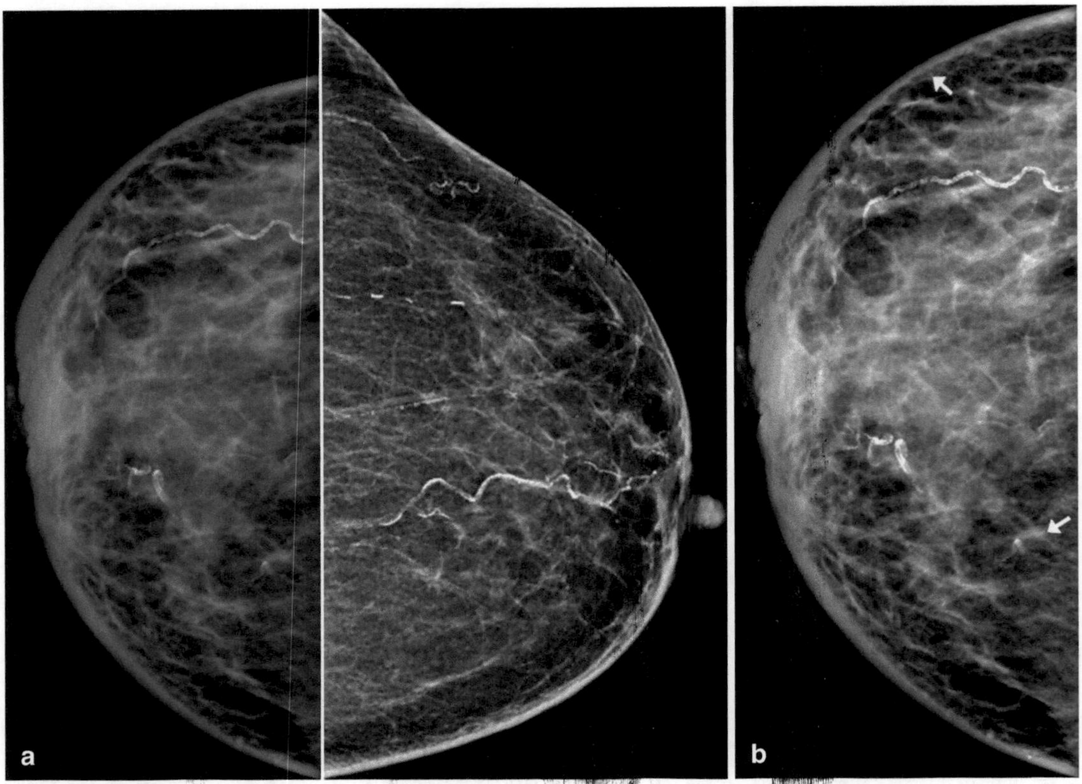

Fig. 5.2 Woman 80 years old with a diagnosis of inflammatory carcinoma (IBC). (**a**) Bilateral mammography in craniocaudal (CC) projection. (**b**) Magnification of right CC projection. The right breast shows thickening and generalized increase of skin density, as well as increase in trabeculation and increase in right breast density, diffuse form (*arrows*)

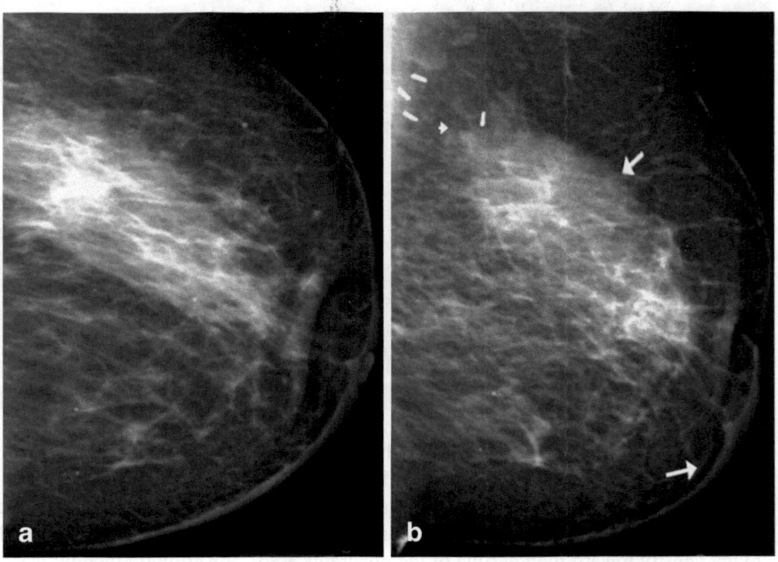

Fig. 5.3 (**a**) Female 54 years of age. Antecedent of conservative surgery with diagnosis of infiltrating ductal carcinoma in left breast. Left mammography in craniocaudal (CC) and mediolateral oblique (MLO) projection. (**b**) Surgical staples are observed toward the upper and lower third quadrant. Skin thickening and retraction (*long arrow*) increase in diffuse CSA mammary density

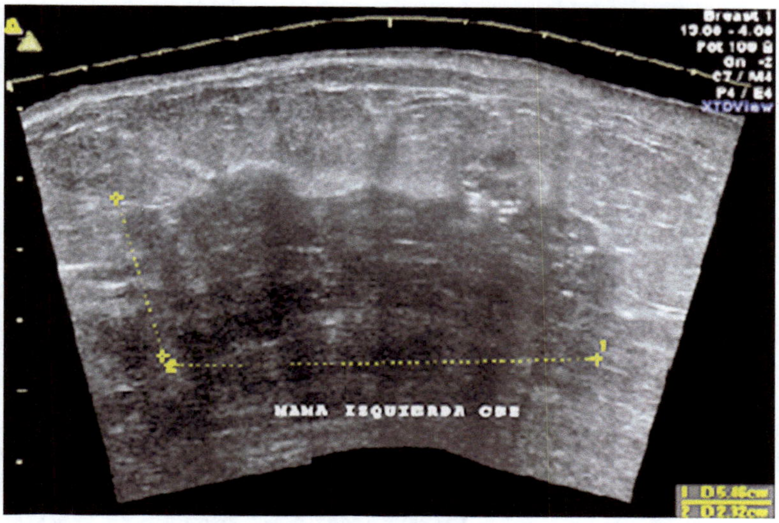

Fig. 5.4 Left breast IBC. Female 57 years of age with a diagnosis of inflammatory carcinoma of the left breast, in extended field of view. In extended field-of-view (EFOV) ultrasound (US), thickening was observed in the skin and heterogenous lymph node tissue; tumors with irregular aspect, solid, hypoechoic, posterior sonic attenuation, associated with breast architecture distortion and thickening of the skin

and digital subtraction, a window could be opened to improvement in diagnosis, principally in localization of the focal lesion and in the extension of the latter.

In contrast, US constitutes an alternative in the detection of IBC without the need for compression or radiation [12].

In multiple reviews, US was superior to mammography in the detection of a primary tumor, this being a key point in the possible differentiation of mastitis, as well as of multifocality or multicentricity. Another advantage of US is that it possesses high sensitivity in the detection of supraclavicular, infraclavicular, or internal mammary chain lymphatic nodes.

Sonographic findings in IC are similar to those present in mastitis or in locally advanced cancer.

Ultrasound

Ultrasound (US) offers an alternative imaging modality for detection, diagnosis, guided biopsy, and evaluation of the response to neoadjuvant chemotherapy in IC without the necessity of compression or ionizing radiation. At the University of Texas MD Anderson Cancer Center (MDACC) in Houston, it was demonstrated that it is possible by US to detect breast tumors with irregular aspect, solid and hypoechoic with well-defined margins and posterior acoustic shadow, and also skin thickening in up to 95 % of patients with inflammatory breast carcinoma (IBC) [1] (Fig. 5.4).

Technically, US should be performed with a high-frequency linear transducer of 7.5 MHz or more. Echographic examination includes evaluation of the skin, mammary tissue, pectoral muscle, and axillary region.

In the case of detecting a primary lesion of the breast, this should be characterized based on the American College of Radiology (ACR) breast imaging lexicon [14]. Color Doppler and pulsated Doppler echography are employed to evaluate tumor and mammary parenchyma vascularity [4, 16].

The diffuse disease with an infiltration pattern is frequently found in patients with IBC; thus, a technique with an EFOV would have to be employed because this would permit a greater appreciation of the disease extension, and, different from mammography, US allows evaluation of axillary, infra-, and supraclavicular lymph nodes and the internal mammary chain [15, 16] (Fig. 5.4).

Sonographic Findings in Inflammatory Breast Cancer

The most frequent sonographic findings include one or multiple mass(es) in >50 %; the most frequent morphology is lobular and irregular with

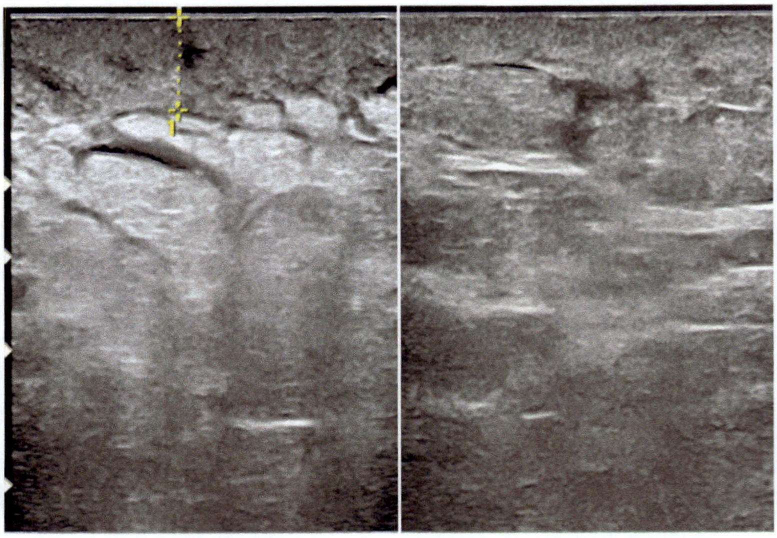

Fig. 5.5 Woman aged 52 years with inflammatory carcinoma of the left breast that shows the skin as hypoechoic, heterogeneous, with loss of interface with subcutaneous tissue, with a maximum thickness of 8 mm and dilated lymph nodes

indistinct or poorly defined borders. The majority of the masses detected measure 2 cm or more.

Skin thickening presents with associated diffuse edema of the subadjacent tissue, thermal emboli, and thermal lymph node affectation; it is observed to be hypoechoic, heterogenous, with >3-mm thickness, and without adequate interface with subcutaneous cell tissue (Fig. 5.5).

Edema and dilation of the lymph node ducts condition a marked hypoechoic and diffuse visualization of the mammary gland tissue.

There are regional lymphadenopathies, and US is the most useful tool for performing biopsies of suspicious lymph nodes and to detect metastatic disease (Fig. 5.6a–c). Axillary adenopathies were predominantly detected, with the ability to detect adenopathies of supraclavicular, infraclavicular, and the internal mammary chain [15, 16].

Microcalcifications are not really detected by US; however, microcalcifications have been detected in the studies of patients with IC. In these cases, mammography continues to be the study with the greatest sensitivity for their detection, associating their presence with multifocality and multicentricity.

Magnetic Resonance

MR of the breast is the imaging tool of choice in the evaluation of patients with IC. Recent studies have analyzed the efficacy of the different imaging modalities in the evaluation of patients with this pathology, finding that the MR modality is more precise for detection in comparison with mammography, with a sensitivity of up to 99 % [1, 17].

Up to 100 % of mammary parenchyma, MR detects alterations in clinically suspicious patients [1, 17].

A 1.5- or 3-T resonator was employed with breast-specific surface bobbins, placing the patient in prone, decubitus position on the table and carrying out the following: 2D diffusion sequences (value *b*: 500 and 1,000 s/mm^2 on axial plane; 2D-FSE potentiated with fat suppression, 2D-S potentiated in T2 with fat suppression, 2D-SE potentiated in T1 on axial plane) and 3D-SPGR pre- and postcontrast intravenous (IV) (gadolinium) with dynamic study [1].

Afterward, the images are studied and worked on at a specific workstation.

The most important findings are thickening of the skin with a diameter >3 mm and reinforcement with greater frequency of irregular focal or diffuse nodular type in 90–100 % [17] (Fig. 5.7).

Fifty percent of patients present associated edema, including prepectoral edema, manifesting as an increase in sequence T2 signal intensity.

There is the presence of unique or multiple nodule(s) distributed in diffuse manner in the breast, with irregular morphology, which can be contiguous because their behavior is iso- or hypointense in the T1 sequence, and in the T1 sequence after administration of contrast, there is

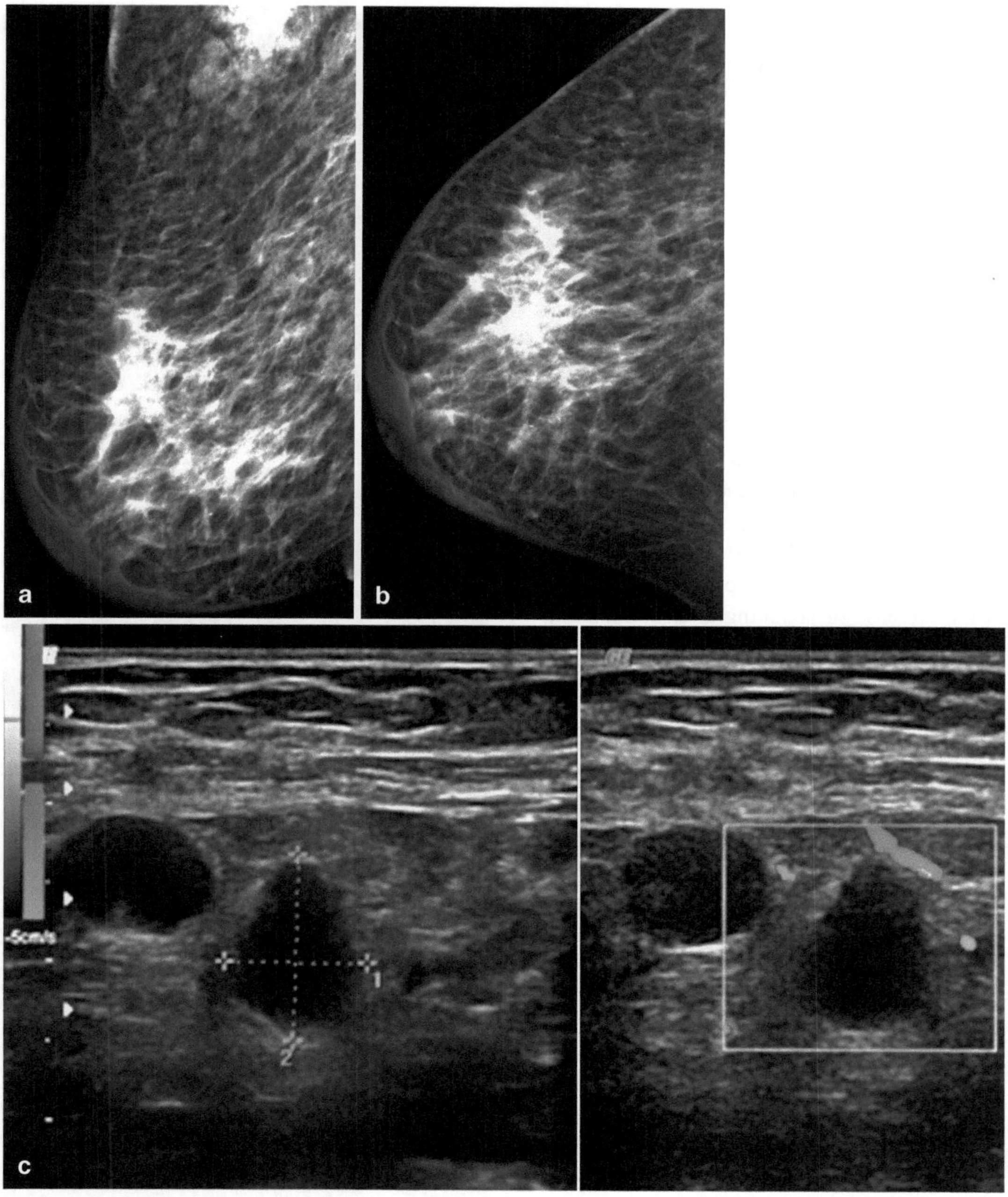

Fig. 5.6 (**a**) Female patient aged 54 years with inflammatory carcinoma (IC) in right breast *mammography*. Craniocaudal (CC) and (**b**) mediolateral oblique view (MLO) projections. Increase in density and trabeculation, generalized thickening of the skin, and the presence of lymph nodes in the ipsilateral region that show a size increase. (**c**) Axillary ultrasound (US) additionally shows cortical thickening and eccentric fatty hilum of the adenomegalies

heterogenous internal reinforcement with variable signal intensity.

In sequence T1 postcontrast (gadolinium), it can also manifest as multiple enhancement regions with fragmented appearance, asymmetrical or patchy; heterogeneous separated by normal or fatty mammary parenchyma zones; and it is unilateral.

The abnormal reinforcement areas present a type III kinetic washout curve or a plateau (delayed reinforcement) type II curve in 97 %,

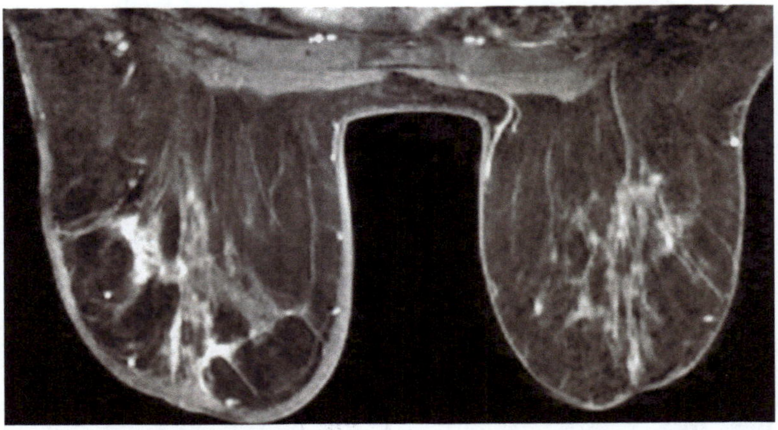

Fig. 5.7 Woman aged 70 years with a diagnosis of inflammatory carcinoma (IC). In axial cut, postcontrast Vibrant, the image shows diffuse thickening of the skin with marked asymmetry in the left breast and multiple nonmass reinforcements in glandular tissue

and in diffusion sequences, restriction of diffuse form is identified with values of ADC variables [1, 18] (Fig. 5.8a, b).

It has been found that the amount and distribution of blood microvessels play an important role in the increase of signaling after administration of paramagnetic contrast because initial rapid reinforcement is associated with neoangiogenesis. The formation of new capillaries in preexisting vessels is an important component that presents in malignant tumors, and preexisting neovascularization is characteristic.

The washout phenomenon is caused by arteriovenous anastomosis with washout and consequent mean exit flow to a great number of capillaries with high-speed arterial flow, resulting in rapid transport of the contrast medium from the intravascular to the interstitial compartment.

Its most frequent localization is dorsal and central, with greater frequency in comparison with granulomatous mastitis, which is predominantly subareolar [1].

In the spectroscopy, a Cho peak of 3.2 ppm was registered. This is useful for assessing treatment response, observing a diminution in the peak [19, 20].

This is useful for assessing chest wall integrity and for discarding infiltration (Fig. 5.9).

Ninety percent present ipsilateral axillary adenopathies and even of the internal mammary chains, identifying lymph nodes with cortical thickening and size increase, as well as loss of morphology, which are better assessed in the short T1 inversion recovery (STIR) sequence [1, 18] (Fig. 5.10a–g).

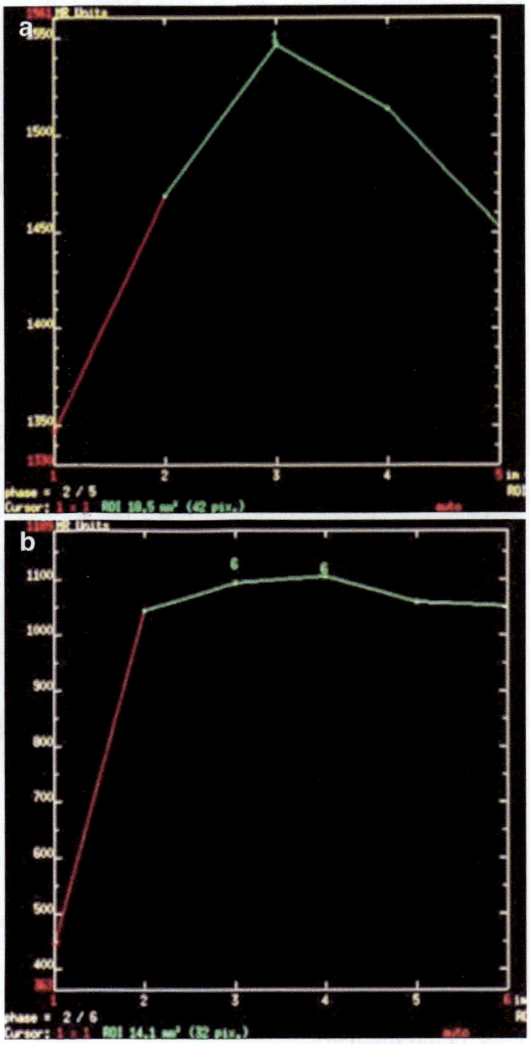

Fig. 5.8 (**a**) Types of enhancement curves assessed by MRI. Type III curve with initial uptake and rapid washout. (**b**) Type II curve with late reinforcement (plateau)

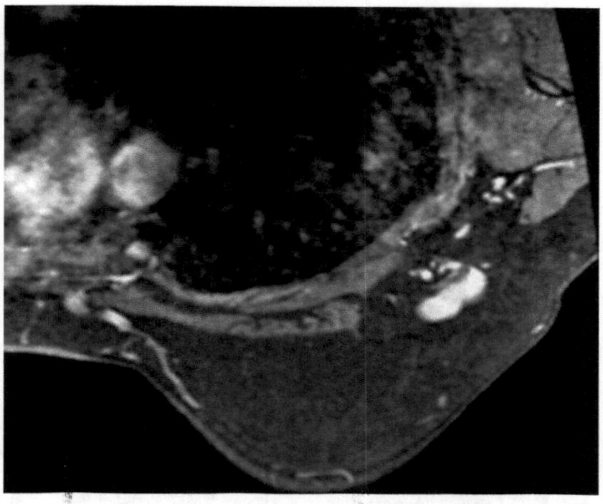

Fig. 5.9 Female, 55 years of age with an antecedent of left breast inflammatory carcinoma, identifying in a short T1 inversion recovery (STIR) sequence MR lymph nodes that show increase in their dimensions as well as infiltration-associated fatty hilum loss

Findings in Nuclear Medicine

Positron emission tomography (PET) is a molecular imaging technique that is sensitive to metabolic changes in the tissues. In these cases, it is utilized as an 18-fluorodeoxyglucose (18FDG)-marked radiotracer, which possesses great affinity in tumor lesions. Simple PET is metabolically useful for detecting tumor lesions >1 cm; however, on fusing PET modalities with (PET/CT), not only is tissue functioning obtained but also their anatomical correlation, which allows assessment of the lesion's extension at the locoregional level as well as at a distance [22].

In the different prospective studies, limited usefulness of PET has been found with 18FDG in small-sized lesions or in early breast cancer stages, while it is mainly useful in assessing local lymph node affectation and distant metastasis; it is not applicable in patients with IC, who frequently have extensive locoregional disease [10].

In a preliminary study of the role of PET-CT with 24 patients with IC, its effectiveness was shown in demonstrating locoregional and distant disease. This study demonstrated multicentric IC in 63 % of patients, regional lymph node affectation in 88 %, and distant metastasis in 38 %, principally affecting liver, bone, and contralateral supraclavicular lymph nodes [10].

The diagnostic efficacy of PET 18FDG in palpable tumors is superior to other imaging techniques. The high positive predictive value (PPV) of PET suggests an important role in the identification of multicentricity of the primary tumor as well as of those at a distance. The radiotracer's uptake pattern will depend on the extension of the carcinoma, showing diffuse or focalized hypermetabolism. It permits us to evaluate the local and the distant state, as well as bone metastases and those of other organs [21, 22].

For diagnosis of IC, hypermetabolism of the affected breast and diffuse hypermetabolic thickening of the skin were found in the patients evaluated [10, 21].

Another usefulness of PET-CT comprises monitoring and assessment of the response of the carcinoma, as well as of the metastases with chemotherapy. Generally, a study is conducted at the beginning and another at the end of treatment; on some occasions, an intermediate follow-up can be intercalated. This method does not replace other imaging studies such as mammography and US; it is a tool to aid in disease follow-up or in doubtful cases or in those with difficult diagnosis [21].

In the study of Yang published in 2007, in which the author analyzes the sensitivity of the mammography, US, MR, and PET-CT in the diagnosis of IC, he found that MR showed 100 % sensitivity, PET-CT 96 %, US 95 %, and mammography 80 %. In this evaluation, the author mentions that mammary density can be a determining factor for the sensitivity of the mammography in this series [1].

A limitation in daily practice is that it is not always possible to perform all of the proposed

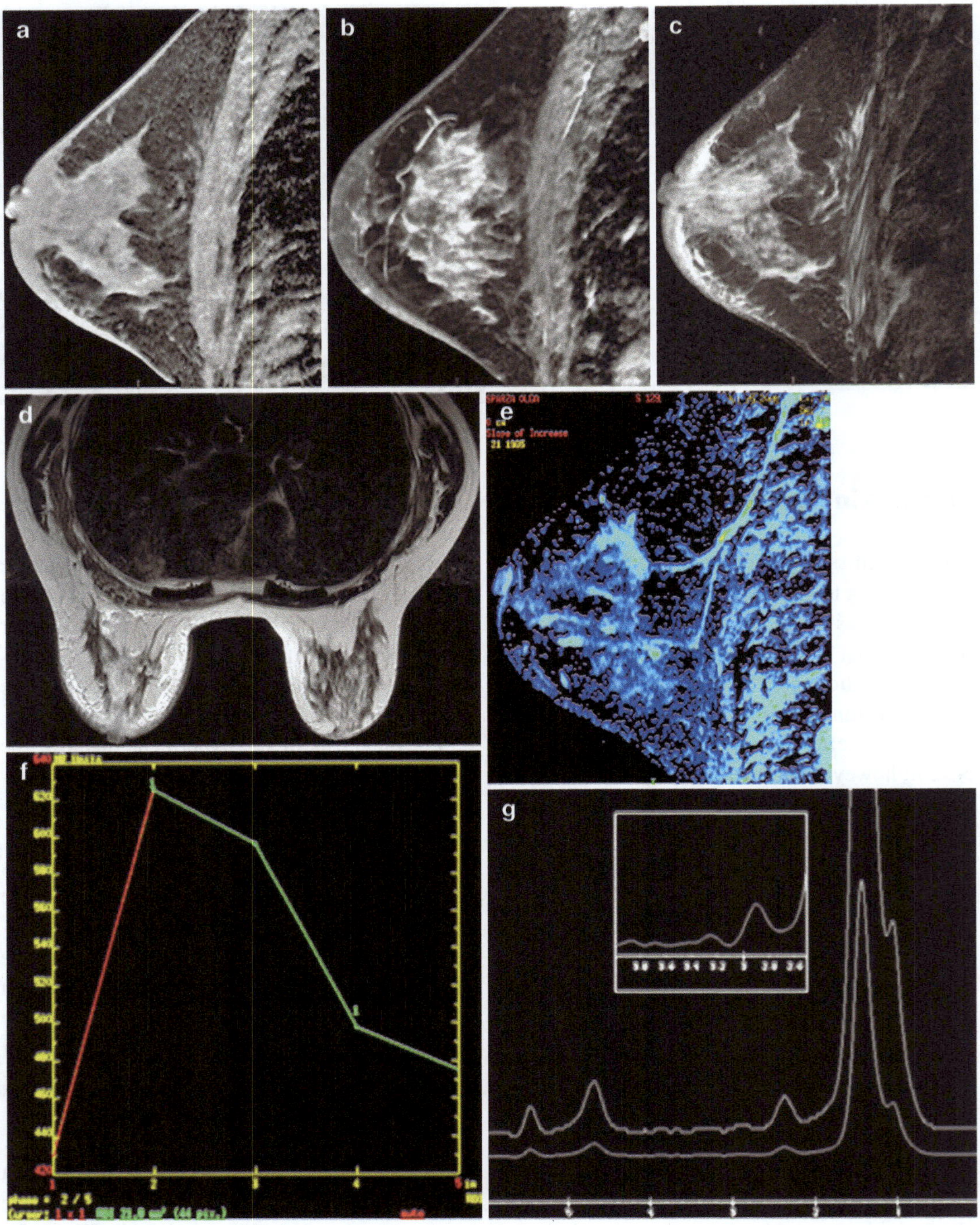

Fig. 5.10 Woman 46 years of age with a diagnosis of inflammatory breast cancer (IBC) that initiated clinically with left breast volume increase, hyperemia, and pain on diagnosis of inflammatory carcinoma (IC). (**a**) The sagittal T1 sequence showed skin thickening with 8-mm thickness of periareolar predominance, with areas of hyperintense distortion with diffuse and contiguous distribution; (**b**) with nonmass reinforcement in T1 sequence with diffuse and heterogenous contrast; and (**c**) prepectoral level hyperintensity in short T1 inversion recovery (STIR), as well as (**d**) central predominant hyperintensity in T2 sequence due to important edema in glandular tissue (**e**) in the color map, uptake zones were observed, (**f**) showing a type III curve (washout) and (**g**) negative spectroscopy

imaging studies on all of the patients, whether due to accessibility or costs, and many women initiate treatment without having a series of complete imaging analyses. Recent MR and PET/CT modalities have been gaining, little by little, an important role in the diagnosis and management of the disease. The Yang study proposes that MR could be the initial imaging modality in suspicious cases of IC, and PET/CT would be an ideal partner for detection of distant metastases [21].

In the study of Jean-Louis Alberini, in which the author evaluated 59 patients with IC, it was found that PET was positive in all patients (100 %), and the primary tumor exhibited a diffuse hypermetabolic pattern in 15 % and a localized pattern in the remainder of cases, among which this was multifocal in 18 patients and unifocal in 32 patients; there were three cases of granulomatous mastitis, which are considered false positives, given that the radiotracer is not specific for cancer [23].

The standardized uptake value $(SUV)_{max}$ is the value that permits measurement of the radiotracer concentration in a determined space or site of interest. This value was high in cases of carcinomas as well as in those of mastitis; thus, it was impossible to differentiate between both entities [23].

Skin-level hypermetabolism was found in 78 % of cases with IC but was not observed in patients with mastitis [5].

On assessing regional lymph nodes, in 89.9 % of cases, focal lymph node uptake presented at the ipsilateral axillary or the extra-axillary level: retropectoral, supra- or infraclavicular, or at that of the internal mammary chain [23].

It is noteworthy that PET or PET-CT with 18 FDG can be altered in patients with diabetes, causing false negatives [5, 23].

In 31 % [18] of cases, distant metastasis was detected, which was corroborated by conventional imaging studies only in 12 cases; affected sites ranged from greater to lesser frequency: in mediastinal, contralateral axillary lymph nodes and in peritoneum and/or ovary. In the cases of metastasis to bone, a lesser sensitivity was observed to scintillography and/or MR [23].

Given the limitation of PET-CT in whole body to detect lesions <1 cm in breast, positron emission mammography (PEM) is being developed at present; it consists of two X-ray images that are placed in parallel form, and these are positioned as in a mammography, which allows for the detection of smaller-sized lesions, with 91 % sensitivity in cases of ductal carcinoma in situ and 89 % in infiltrating cancer. With regard to inflammatory cancer, given that this is a very recent technology, its usefulness is currently being investigated [22] (Fig. 5.11).

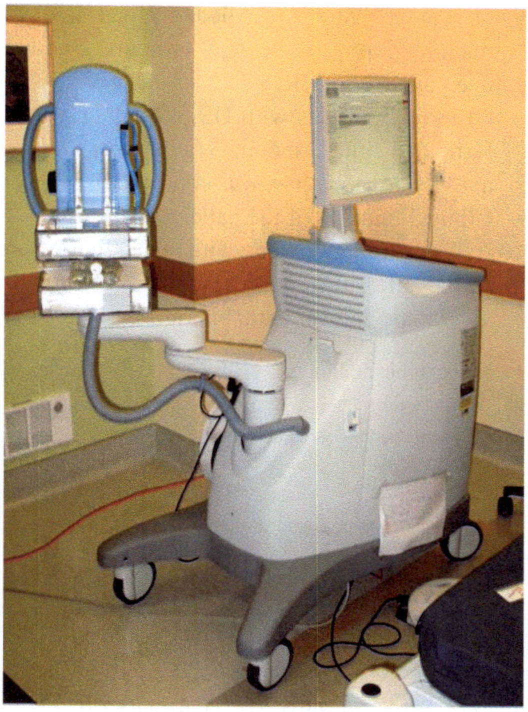

Fig. 5.11 Positron emission mammography (PEM) equipment

The Mexican city-based Instituto Nacional de Cancerología-México (INCan) is conducting a 4-year retrospective review from January 2007 to October 2011 in 84 patients with clinical suspicion of inflammatory carcinoma, confirming this in 54 patients with a histopathologic study:

- Average age at time of diagnosis was 51.4 years (range, 33–91 years).
- Left breast was the more affected one, with 26 cases; right breast with 22 cases; and both breasts, two patients.

- Of the 50 patients studied, 37 had US, 42 mammography, three had tomography, and one patient had MR.
- Of the 37 patients with US, 33 demonstrated skin thickening, and in 31, the presence of axillary adenopathies was confirmed.
- Clinical findings of the patients were:
  - There is agreement with that reported in the literature with respect to mammographic and sonographic findings.

Mammographic finding	Patients
Nipple retraction	8
Microcalcifications associated with an increase in density	5
Skin thickening	14
Trabecular and stromal alterations	16

References

1. Yang WT, Le-Petross HT, Macapinlac H, et al. Inflammatory breast cancer: PET/CT, MRI, mammography, and sonography findings. Breast Cancer Res Treat. 2008;109:417–26.
2. Edge SB, Byrd DR, Compton CC, et al. AJCC cancer staging manual. 7th ed. New York: Springer; 2010.
3. Bonnier P, Charpin C, et al. Inflammatory carcinomas of the breast a clinical, pathological, or a clinical and pathological definition? Int J Cancer. 1995;62:382–5.
4. Le-Petross H, Uppendahl L, Stafford J. Sonographic features of inflammatory breast cancer. Semin Roentgenol. 2011;46(4):275–9.
5. Haagensen C. Diseases of the breast. 2ath ed. Philadelphia: Pasauder; 1971. p. 569–84.
6. Kim T, Lau J, Erban J. Lack of uniform diagnostic criteria for inflammatory breast cancer limits interpretation of treatment outcomes: a systematic review. Clin Breast Cancer. 2006;7:386–95. CrossRefMedlineWeb of Science.
7. Kushwaha AC, Whitman GJ, Stelling CB, Cristofanilli MC, Buzdar AU. Primary inflammatory carcinoma of the breast: retrospective review of mammographic findings. AJR Am J Roentgenol. 2000;174:535–8.
8. Tardivon AA, Viala J, Rudelli AC, Guinebretiere JM, Vanel D. Mammographic patterns of inflammatory breast carcinoma: a retrospective study of 92 cases. Eur J Radiol. 1997;24:124–30.
9. Buzdar AU, et al. Effectiveness of mastectomy. Cancer. 1995;76:2286–2290.
10. Yang WT. Advances in imaging of inflammatory breast cancer. Cancer. 2010;116:2755–7.
11. Lee KW, Chung SY, Yang I, et al. Inflammatory breast cancer imaging findings. J Clin Imaging. 2005;29:22–5.
12. Günhan-Bilgen I, Ustun EE, Memis A. Inflammatory breast carcinoma: mammographic, ultrasonographic, clinical, and pathologic findings in 142 cases. Radiology. 2002;223:829–38.
13. Robertson FM, Bondy M, Yang W, et al. Inflammatory breast cancer. The disease, the biology, the treatment. CA Cancer J Clin. 2010;60:351–75.
14. American College of Radiology (ACR). Illustrated breast imaging reporting and data system (BI-RADS). 3rd ed. Reston: American College of Radiology; 1998. p. 121–39.
15. Huong T, Le-Petross HT, Cristofanilli M, Carkaci S, Krishnamurthy S. MRI features of inflammatory breast cancer. AJR Am J Roentgenol. 2011;197(4): 769–76.
16. Sirishma Kalli S, Freer PE, Elizabeth A, Rafferty EA. 16 Lesions of the skin and superficial tissue at breast MR imaging. Radiographics. 2010;30:1891–913.
17. Renz DM, Baltzer PAT, Böttcher J, Thaher F, Gajda M, Camara O, Runnebaum IB, Kaiser WA. Magnetic resonance imaging of inflammatory breast carcinoma and acute mastitis. A comparative study. Eur Radiol. 2008;18:2370–80.
18. Le-Petross HT, Cristofanilli M, Carkaci S, Krishnamurthy S. MRI features of inflammatory breast cancer. AJR. 2011;197(4):769–76.
19. Thukral A, Thomasson DM, Chow CK, Eulate R, Wedam SB. Inflammatory breast cancer: dynamic contrast-enhanced MR in patients receiving bevacizumab- initial experience 1. Radiology. 2007;244(3): 727–35.
20. Martincich L, Montemurro F, De Rosa G, Marra V, Ponzone R, Cirillo S, Gatti M. Monitoring response to primary chemotherapy in breast cancer using dynamic contrast-enhanced magnetic resonance imaging. Breast Cancer Res Treat. 2004;83:67–76.
21. Muna M, Siema B, Bakheet M, et al. 18-Fluorodeoxyglucose-positron emission tomography in inflammatory breast cancer. World J Surg. Société Internationale de Chirurgie. 2003;27(10):1099–104.
22. Robertson FM, Bondy M, et al. Inflammatory breast cancer. The disease, the biology, the treatment. CA Cancer J Clin. 2010;60:351–75.
23. AlberiniJ-L,LerebourѕL,etal.18F-fluorodeoxyglucose positron emission tomography/computed tomography (FDG-PET/CT) imaging in the staging and prognosis of inflammatory breast cancer. Cancer. 2009;115: 5038–47.

Chemotherapy in Inflammatory Breast Cancer

6

Claudia Arce-Salinas, Flavia Morales-Vasquez, Fernando Lara-Medina, and Silvia Patricia Villarreal-Colin

Summary

Historically, survival of patients with inflammatory breast cancer (IBC) has been poor, ranging from only 2.4 months to 26 months from the time of diagnosis to death [1]. Surgery was the first treatment modality employed for IBC; however, all patients developed systemic disease. Kell and Morrow [2] reported an average 5-year overall survival (OS) rate of 4 % in 293 patients with IBC treated with mastectomy with or without radiation. Also, surgery alone results in local recurrence rates of approximately 50 %; this local recurrence was associated with mean survival of <2 years [3]. At present, another strategy comprises the use of molecular and genetic management.

Antecedents

Since 1970, chemotherapy was introduced as a primary treatment for IBC. The addition of chemotherapy (CT) followed sequentially by surgery and radiation resulted in an improvement in disease-free survival (DFS) and OS for patients with this aggressive form of breast cancer, as compared with historical controls [4, 5]. However, local recurrence occurred in 25–39 % of cases despite of the combination of CT, surgery, and radiotherapy (RT), without benefit in survival [6].

In 1977, the Mexican experience in the treatment of IBC was published by De la Garza et al. [7]. These authors treated 18 patients between the years 1970 and 1976 with preoperative CT based on weekly 5-fluorouracil (5-FU) during 2 months, followed by RT, surgery, and CT for 2 years. Over-all response (OR) (complete and partial) was achieved in 16 patients, and median survival for patients with complete response (CR) was 39.3 and 20.6 months for those with partial response (PR). After 72 months of follow-up, four patients were alive [4, 5].

Israel et al. [8] treated 25 patients with IBC between 1978 and 1983 with three cycles of 5-FU and cyclophosphamide followed by surgery and the same CT regimen for 2 years. Overall clinical response was 96 % (two CR and 22 PR). Local relapse was presented in 53.8 % of cases, and median DFS was 45 months.

Usefulness of Chemoimmunotherapy

Based on experimental protocols consisting of bacterial vaccines or nonspecific immunostimulants that demonstrated tumor regression of transplanted, syngeneic hepatocarcinoma grown in guinea pigs and elimination of regional lymph node metastases in the majority of animals after injection of viable

C. Arce-Salinas, M.D., M.Sc. (✉) • F. Morales-Vasquez, M.D., M.S. • F. Lara-Medina, M.D. • S.P. Villarreal-Colin, M.D.
Department of Medical Oncology, Instituto Nacional de Cancerologia-Mexico, Ave. San Fernando 22, Tlalpan, Mexico City, DF 14480, Mexico
e-mail: haydee.arce96@gmail.com

J.G. de la Garza-Salazar et al. (eds.), *Inflammatory Breast Cancer*, DOI 10.1007/978-0-85729-991-8_6,

bacille Calmette-Guérin (BCG) [9], this strategy was incorporated into breast cancer treatment. The concept generated was "systemic cell-mediated tumor immunity" and was demonstrated by rapid rejection of a second tumor challenge several weeks after BCG treatment [10].

In a trial conducted at the MD Anderson Cancer Center in Houston, Texas, USA [4] with 32 patients treated between 1973 and 1977 with IBC, these received three or four cycles of doxorubicin, fluorouracil, and cyclophosphamide without systemic therapy; at the end of RT, patients continued with the same CT regimen until reaching the total dose of 450 mg/m^2 of doxorubicin. After this, patients continued with fluorouracil and cyclophosphamide for up to 2 years, and their treatment was combined with BCG vaccination. Patients were compared with historical controls treated with RT alone. The median DFS interval was 9 months for the irradiation group and 22.8 months for the combined modality group ($p = 0.002$). Nine patients (28 %) in the combined modality group were alive and disease-free with follow-up ranging from 42 to 76 months. In the irradiation group, only two patients (6 %) have remained disease-free at 47 and 57 months, the overall survival of both groups. OS was 30 months for the combined modality group versus 18 months for the control group, with an absolute benefit of 12 months ($p = 0.009$). Subgroup analysis shows that women aged >50 years demonstrated an improvement at 24 months (42 vs. 18 months, respectively) ($p = 0.003$).

In a trial carried out by Zylberberg et al. [7], 15 patients with IBC were treated with doxorubicin, vincristine, cyclophosphamide, 5-FU, and melphalan every 28 days in combination with BCG for three cycles, followed by radical mastectomy and the same CT regimen for ten cycles. Patients also received RT 42 Gy and a 20-Gy boost. BCG was administered for 3 years. All patients had clinical response and three of these, CR. At 56 months of follow-up, median survival was not achieved.

In a small trial performed by Weissman et al. [11], 13 patients with IBC were treated with CT, 5-fluorouracil, doxorubicin, and cyclophosphamide (FAC); mastectomy; and immunotherapy utilizing irradiated allogeneic breast cancer cells admixed with BCG and adjuvant CMV. The authors reported that there was complete eradication of the detectable tumor in 3 of 11 operative specimens (pathologic complete response, pCR). At a median follow-up time of 21 months, only seven patients received homogenous treatment, two of these experienced disease relapse.

These results of these small trials initially supported the use of doxorubicin and BCG; however, due to the lack of specificity and the same results without BCG, this modality was abandoned.

Use of Anthracyclines

Ueno et al. [12] reviewed the outcome of 178 patients with IBC treated with a variety of combined modality approaches at the MD Anderson Cancer Center over the past 20 years. Each protocol included induction CT, then local therapy (RT or mastectomy), then adjuvant CT, and, if mastectomy was performed, adjuvant RT. CT consisted of FAC with or without vincristine and prednisone (VP). In protocol D, patients received an alternate adjuvant CT regimen, methotrexate and vinblastine (MV), if they did not have a CR to induction CT. Median follow-up was 21–45 months according to each protocol. An estimated 28 % of patients were currently disease-free beyond 15 years. Among initial recurrences, 20 % of patients had local failure, 39 % systemic failure, and 9 % central nervous system (CNS) recurrence. Initial response to induction CT was an important prognostic factor. DFS at 15 years was 44 % in patients who had CR to induction CT, 31 % in those with PR, and 7 % in those who had less than PR. There was no improvement in OS or DFS among patients who underwent alternate CT (MV) compared with those who did not.

Chevalier et al. [13] treated 45 women with newly diagnosed IBC with an intensive neoadjuvant CT regimen comprising 5-fluorouracil, epirubicin, and cyclophosphatase high dose [FEC-HD] repeated every 21 days, followed by surgery or RT. After at least two cycles, these patients exhibited disappearance of inflammatory signs in 91 % and improvement in the remaining 9 % of patients. There were 13 (28.9 %) clinical CR, 30 (66.6 %) PR, and two (4.5 %) without change and without progression. After induction CT, modified radical mastectomy was performed in 39 patients, and treatment comprised RT alone in six. pCR was found in ten cases (25.6 %). Hematologic toxicity was grade 4, and neutropenia was observed at day 14 in 100 % of patients. No toxic death occurred. An update of this analysis with 10 years of follow-up and including 120 patients reported that DFS and OS rates were 35.7 % and 41.2 %, respectively. Five patients developed a temporary decrease in left ventricular ejection fraction without congestive heart failure [14].

Another French phase II trial [15] evaluated the combination of 5-FU, doxorubicin, and cyclophosphamide (FAC) in 43 patients with IBC. After three chemotherapy cycles, responding patients underwent surgery. CT was then completed for nine cycles of FAC followed by locoregional RT. Concurrent tamoxifen 40 mg/day was administered for 1 year from time of diagnosis. Thirty-eight patients (88 %) had clinical response to CT and underwent surgery. With a median 48-month follow-up, the predicted 5-year DFS was 48 %.

The conclusions of these trials were that anthracycline treatment was effective in converting inoperable into operable tumors and in improving DFS and local control [16]. However, optimal CT duration and optimal local control (RT and surgery) remain unsolved.

The Taxanes

Another attempt to improve the prognosis of IBC was the introduction of new drugs. Taxanes had shown benefit in metastatic breast cancer. In IBC, a trial conducted at the MD Anderson Cancer Center [17] included 44 patients treated with induction CT (FAC for four cycles), mastectomy, adjuvant CT, and RT, and preoperative paclitaxel for patients with less than PR. A result shows that 34 patients (81 %) achieved objective clinical remission. Six patients (14 %) achieved pathologic complete remission. Sixteen patients were treated with paclitaxel; seven of these (44 %) were able to undergo mastectomy. Median time to progression (TTP) was 22 months, and median OS was 46 months.

The German Preoperative Adriamycin Docetaxel Group (GeparTrio) trial [18] randomized 93 patients with IBC to receive six or eight cycles of Taxotere (docetaxel), Adriamycin (doxorubicin), and Cytoxan (cyclophosphamide) (TAC) or two cycles of TAC, then four cycles of vinorelbine/capecitabine. This group of patients was compared with 194 patients with locally advanced breast cancer (LABC) and 1,777 patients with operable disease. The main objective of this trial was to evaluate pCR. No difference was found between CT regimens, and pCR was achieved in 8.6 % of patients. In Table 6.1, summarized are the recent neoadjuvant trials done in IBC.

High-Dose Chemotherapy

The use of multimodality treatment regimens has improved survival rates over treatment with RT or surgery alone or combined, but the 5-year DFS rate for patients with IBC currently remains at only approximately 30 %. In an attempt to achieve higher rates of CR and survival, the use of high-dose chemotherapy (HDCT) supported by autologous stem cell transplantation (ASCT) as a component of multimodality therapy regimens has been evaluated. Several small phase II trials conducted during the 1990s suggested that HDCT yields survival benefits for patients with high-risk or metastatic breast cancer, including IBC [23]. Our impression at the present time is that ASCT is not recommended.

A trial was carried out by Adkins et al. [24] between 1989 and 1997, in which he included 47 patients with IBC. These were treated with HDCT. Neoadjuvant and adjuvant CT were administered to 33 and 34 patients, respectively, and 20 patients received both. All patients received HDCT with ASCT, and 41 patients received locoregional RT. Mean follow-up was 30 months. DFS and OS from diagnosis were 57.7 % and 59.1 %, respectively.

Table 6.1 Summary of the most recent neoadjuvant trials in IBC

Author	Patients (*n*)	Chemotherapy	Response rate (%)	Median survival (months)
Cristofanilli [17]	44	FEC-T	81	46
De Boer [16]	54	EC followed by 5-FU (infusion)	79	23
Harris [19]	54	CAM/FAC	30	62
Cristofanilli [20]	240	FAC vs. FAC-T	74 vs. 82 %	OS 32 vs. 54 (p=0.003)
Low [21]	46	CAM +/– FU +/– tam	NA	OS 3.8 years EFS 2.3 years
Evans [22]	53	AC vs. AD	61 vs. 71 % ns	NA

FAC fluorouracil/adriamycin/cyclophosphamide, *T* paclitaxel, *tam* tamoxifen, *EC* epirubicin/ cyclophosphamide, *CAM* cyclophosphamide/adriamycin/methotrexate, *AC* Adriamycin/ cyclophosphamide, *AD* adriamycin/docetaxel, *NA* not applicable, *OS* overall survival, *EFS* event-free survival, *NS* not significant

Table 6.2 Trials with HDCT in IBC

Author	Patients (*n*)	HDCT	MS	OS
Schwartzberg [27]	56	CTCb	NA	At 3 years, 75 %
Viens [28]	100	Sequential HDCT with CDF	NA	At 3 years, 70 %
Arun [29]	24	Escalating carboplatin/ cyclophosphamide	NA	At 2 years, 73 %
Smlo [26]	120	Several regimens used in single or tandem DICT	NA	At 5 years, 64 %
Bertucci [30]	74	Conventional anthracycline-based SDCT vs. HDCT (cyclophosphamide/ melphalan/methotrexate)	NA	18 % vs. 50 %

CDF cyclophosphamide/doxorubicin/5-fluorouracil, *CTCb* cyclophosphamide/thiotepa/carboplatin, *DICT* dose-intensive chemotherapy, *HDCT* high-dose chemotherapy, *NA* not available, *MS* median survival, *OS* overall survival, *yrs.* years, *SDCT* standard dose chemotherapy

Cagnoni et al. [25] included 30 patients from 1993 to 1997; there were 30 patients with IBC. Twenty-three patients received neoadjuvant chemotherapy (NAC) prior to HDCT; 18 patients also received adjuvant CT following surgery but prior to HDC. All patients received HDC with high-dose cyclophosphamide, cisplatin, and carmustine (bis-chloroethylnitrosourea, BCNU) with progenitor cell support. Every patient underwent surgery. Patients received RT after HDC in addition to tamoxifen if their tumors were estrogen receptor (ER) positive. Results showed than 40 % of patients presented drug-induced injury; in addition, one toxic death was reported. Median follow-up was 23.5 months, and DFS was 70 %.

One of the larger nonrandomized studies of HDCT in IBC was conducted by Somlo et al. [26], who administered postoperative, dose-intensive CT to patients with IBC as part of a late-stage treatment intensification strategy. The authors included 120 patients, who were treated with induction CT consisting of anthracycline and/or taxanes prior to undergoing surgery. The patients then received sequentially developed, single, or tandem dose-intensive CT with one of several different regimens. At a median follow-up of 61 months, estimated 5-year relapse-free survival and OS rates were 44 and 64 %, respectively. The authors found that ER/ progesterone receptor (PR) status and degree of lymph node involvement were the best predictors of response. In Table 6.2, we find a summary of the most common HDCT trials.

HDCT improves OS; however, there are small trials with the lack of a control group. Additional studies are necessary to establish the role of this treatment.

Conclusions

In conclusion, multimodality treatment is the standard of treatment for IBC, and induction CT followed by surgery and RT comprises the best sequence. However, for this good result to be achieved, more efforts are required to improve prognosis, such as the use of targeted therapy.

References

1. Wang CC, Griscom NT. Inflammatory carcinoma of the breast. Results following orthovoltage and supervoltage radiation therapy. Clin Radiol. 1964;15: 167–74.
2. Kell MR, Morrow M. Surgical aspects of inflammatory breast cancer. Breast Dis. 2005;22:67–73.
3. Bozzetti F, Saccozzi R, De Lena M, Salvadori B. Inflammatory cancer of the breast: analysis of 114 cases. J Surg Oncol. 1981;18:355–61.
4. De la Garza J, de la Huerta R, Torres R, Sánchez-Basurto C. Different management of inflammatory carcinoma, ASCO Meeting. Denver; 1977 Abstract C-32.
5. De la Garza J. Cáncer inflamatorio de la glándula mamaria. Experiencia de 6 años con QT. RT. Cir Ciruj. 1977;45(6):351–7.
6. Barker JL, Montague E, Peters LJ. Clinical experience with irradiation of inflammatory carcinoma of the breast with or without elective chemotherapy. Cancer. 1980;45:625–9.
7. Zytherberg B, Salat-Baroux J, Ravina JH, et al. Intial Chemoimmunotheropy in inflammatory cancinoma of the breast cancer 1982:IS:1537-43
8. Israel L, Breau JL, Morere JF. Two years of high-dose cyclophosphamide and 5-fluorouracil followed by surgery after 3 months for acute inflammatory breast carcinomas. A phase II study of 25 cases with a median follow-up of 35 months. Cancer. 1986;57:24–8.
9. Hanna MG, Zbar B, Rapp HJ. Histopathology of tumor regression after intralesional injection of mycobacterium bovis. I. Tumor growth and metastases. J Natl Cancer Inst. 1972;48:1441–55.
10. Zbar B, Tanaka T. Immunotherapy of cancer: regression of tumors after intralesional injection of *Mycobacterium bovis*. Science. 1971;772:271–3.
11. Wiseman C, Jessup JM, Smith TL, et al. Inflammatory breast cancer treated with surgery, chemotherapy and allogeneic tumor CelVBCG immunotherapy. Cancer. 1982;49:1266–71.
12. Ueno NT, Buzdar AU, Singletary SE, et al. Combined-modality treatment of inflammatory breast carcinoma: twenty years of experience at MD Anderson cancer center. Cancer Chemother Pharmacol. 1997;40:321–9.
13. Chevallier B, Roche H, Olivier JP, et al. Inflammatory breast cancer. Pilot study of intensive induction chemotherapy (FEC-HD) results in a high histologic response rate. Am J Clin Oncol. 1993;16: 223–8.
14. Veyret C, Levy CH, Chollet PH, et al. Inflammatory breast cancer outcome with epirubicin-based induction and maintenance chemotherapy. Ten-year results from the French Adjuvant Study Group GETIS 02 trial. Cancer. 2006;107:2535–44.
15. Maloisel F, Dufour P, Bergerat JP, et al. Results of initial doxorubicin, 5-fluorouracil, and cyclophosphamide combination chemotherapy for inflammatory carcinoma of the breast. Cancer. 1990;65:851–5.
16. De Boer RH, Allum WH, Ebbs SR, et al. Multimodality therapy in inflammatory breast cancer: is there a place for surgery? Ann Oncol. 2000;11:1147–53.
17. Cristofanilli M, Buzdar AU, Sneige N, et al. Paclitaxel in the multimodality treatment for inflammatory breast carcinoma. Cancer. 2001;92:1775–82.
18. Dan Costa S, Sibylle L, Kaufmann M, et al. Neoadjuvant chemotherapy shows similar response in patients with inflammatory or locally advanced breast cancer when compared with operable breast cancer: a secondary analysis of the GeparTrio trial data. J Clin Oncol. 2009;28:83–91.
19. Harris EE, Schultz D, Bertsch H, et al. Ten-year outcome after combined modality therapy for inflammatory breast cancer. Int J Radiat Oncol Biol Phys. 2003;55:1200–8.
20. Cristofanilli M, González-Angulo AM, Buzdar AU, et al. Paclitaxel improves the prognosis in estrogen receptor negative inflammatory breast cancer: the MD Anderson cancer center experience. Clin Breast Cancer. 2004;4:415–9.
21. Low JA, Berman AW, Steinberg SM, et al. Long-term follow-up for locally advanced and inflammatory breast cancer patients treated with multimodality therapy. J Clin Oncol. 2004;22:4067–74.
22. Evans TR, Yellowlees A, Foster E, et al. Phase III randomized trial of doxorubicin and docetaxel versus doxorubicin and cyclophosphamide as primary medical therapy in women with breast cancer: an Anglo Celtic Cooperative Oncology Group study. J Clin Oncol. 2005;23:2988–95.
23. Yang CH, Cristofanilli M. Systemic treatments for inflammatory breast cancer. Breast Dis. 2005;22: 55–65.
24. Adkins D, Brown R, Trinkaus K, et al. Outcomes of high-dose chemotherapy and autologous stem-cell transplantation in stage IIIB inflammatory breast cancer. J Clin Oncol. 1999;17:2006–14.
25. Cagnoni PJ, Nieto Y, Shpall E, et al. High-dose chemotherapy with autologous hematopoietic progenitor-cell support as part of combined modality therapy in patients with inflammatory breast cancer. J Clin Oncol. 1998;16:1661–8.
26. Somlo G, Frankel P, Chow W, et al. Prognostic indicators and survival in patients with stage IIIB inflammatory breast carcinoma after dose-intense chemotherapy. J Clin Oncol. 2004;22:1839–48.
27. Schwartzberg L, Weaver C, Lewkow L, et al. High-dose chemotherapy with peripheral blood stem

cell support for stage IIIB inflammatory carcinoma of the breast. Bone Marrow Transplant. 1999; 24:981–7.

28. Viens P, Palangie T, Janvier M, et al. First-line high-dose sequential chemotherapy with rG-CSF and repeated blood stem cell transplantation in untreated inflammatory breast cancer: toxicity and response (PEGASE 02 trial). Br J Cancer. 1999;81: 449–56.
29. Arun B, Slack R, Gehan E, et al. Survival after autologous hematopoietic stem cell transplantation for patients with inflammatory breast carcinoma. Cancer. 1999;85:93–9.
30. Bertucci F, Tarpin C, Charafe-Jauffret E, et al. Multivariate analysis of survival in inflammatory breast cancer: impact of intensity of chemotherapy in multimodality treatment. Bone Marrow Transplant. 2004;33:913–20.

Radiotherapy in Inflammatory Breast Cancer

7

Diana Vanesa Toledano-Cuevas, Aida Mota-Garcia, and Roque Alberto Guadarrama-Fleites

Introduction

Inflammatory breast cancer (IBC) is an uncommon disease with a poor prognosis reported historically. Clinically, IBC is characterized by erythema and edema of the skin of the breast, called *peau d'orange*, or without an associated palpable mass. Infiltration of dermal lymph nodes is often observed, but its records are not necessary for diagnosis of inflammatory carcinoma.

Despite advances in medical, surgical, and radiation oncology, IBC remains a therapeutic challenge. More than 70 % of patients with IBC have clinically localized disease without distant metastases at initial presentation; thus, they are candidates for potentially curative combined-modality treatments. Locoregional recurrence in this disease is invariably associated with distant dissemination and death [1].

Fortunately the treatment for patients with IBC has evolved significantly over the past decades, incorporating surgery, radiotherapy (RT), and chemotherapy (CT) for local and distant disease control. Although no standard treatment has been defined for this disease [2].

In patients treated with RT alone, with or without CT, the 5-year survival rates are only 5–15 %. In patients treated with surgery and RT, survival rates were similar at 0–20 % [3]. In patients treated with CT in whom good partial or complete clinical response is achieved, one study has questioned whether mastectomy is required in addition to breast and regional nodal irradiation. Other series have shown that the addition of mastectomy to chemoradiation improves local control and, in patients with an objective response to CT, also improves disease-free survival (DFS) [4].

Initially, radiation was used alone, but after systemic treatment became available, neoadjuvant CT followed by mastectomy and radiation became the standard [5]. With improvements in systemic treatment, locoregional management became a critical component in curative treatment. Several studies have found an association between locoregional control (LRC) and overall survival (OS) in patients with IBC treated with CT [6, 7].

The addition of neoadjuvant CT to the treatment regimen made mastectomy an appropriate treatment option for the majority of patients and proved to be a significant therapeutic advance in locoregional management. With the addition of mastectomy, the dose for the twice-daily fractionation scheme was reduced to 45 Gy delivered over 3 weeks, with a 15-Gy boost to the chest wall [8]. An analysis of the first 61 patients with clinically diagnosed IBC who were treated at MD Anderson Cancer Center in Houston, Texas, using this trimodality approach was published in 1989 [9]. This study showed that the initial clinical response to CT was associated with improved 5-year actuarial DFS, and the initial clinical response to CT

D.V. Toledano-Cuevas, M.D. (✉)
A. Mota-Garcia, M.D. • R.A. Guadarrama-Fleites, M.D.
Department of Radiation Oncology, Instituto Nacional de Cancerologia-Mexico, San Fernando N 22, Tlalpan, Mexico City, DF 14080, Mexico
e-mail: dovotoco@yahoo.com.mx

J.G. de la Garza-Salazar et al. (eds.), *Inflammatory Breast Cancer*,
DOI 10.1007/978-0-85729-991-8_7, © Springer-Verlag London 2013

also correlated with the probability of LRC. Five-year actuarial LRC rates were 89 % in patients experiencing complete response (CR), 68 % in those with partial response (PR), and 33 % in those with no response; the overall rate was 58 %. The majority of local failures occurred in the irradiated volume of the chest wall and took place more frequently among patients who did not achieve brisk erythema or moist desquamation from the radiation. In the 46 patients who completed treatment as initially planned (excluding the 9 patients who had immediate postmastectomy radiation secondary to positive margins), no difference in local control was noted between the two radiation fractionation schedules, with 3 of 14 patients (21 %) treated daily and 7 of 32 patients (22 %) treated twice daily failing locally. Because locoregional recurrence in both arms was high, these results provided the rationale for conducting dose-escalation studies employing the twice-daily fractionation scheme.

To evaluate the effects of dose escalation, a specific comparison was made between the 32 patients who were treated postmastectomy with twice-daily radiation at a total dose of 60 Gy and the 39 patients who were treated similarly but at a total dose of 66 Gy. There was significant improvement in LRC in the higher-dose group compared with the lower-dose group, that is, 84 versus 58 % and 77 versus 58 % at 5 and 10 years, respectively ($p=0.04$). A statistically significant improvement also occurred in 5- and 10-year OS rates between these two groups ($p=0.03$), and a trend toward improvement in 5- and 10-year DFS rates was noted ($p=0.06$). As also noted in other studies, the degree of initial response to CT significantly predicted better local control, OS, and DFS. Patients whose disease did not respond to CT had extremely poor outcomes regardless of treatment, with 5-year OS and DFS rates of 9 and 3 %, respectively. Late toxicity occurred in 23 patients (20 %). This complication rate was similar in patients treated prior to and after 1986 [9].

In the literature, the role of surgery in IBC has been controversial. In the, to our knowledge, only prospective randomized study comparing surgery vs. RT following neoadjuvant CT, in 57 patients with IBC, Mourali et al. [10] did not find any significant difference in DFS between the two groups. De Boer et al. [11] found no differences in OS, DFS, and disease-free relapse in a retrospective comparison between two groups of patients with IBC: one treated with surgery and RT and the other with RT alone after neoadjuvant CT. But patients with CCR were encouraged to have RT alone. In the MD Anderson trial in 178 patients, the authors found that patients who exhibited a response to induction CT benefitted from the addition of mastectomy to treatment comprising CT and radiation [8, 12].

A major advance in the last three decades has been the introduction of a multidisciplinary approach to the management of this aggressive disease, incorporating preoperative chemotherapy, surgery, and radiation therapy; this approach has significantly improved survival [13].

Preoperative Radiotherapy

Patients with adequate response after neoadjuvant CT and with operable disease are submitted to radical mastectomy 3–4 weeks after the completion of CT, and those with inoperable disease should receive CT with methotrexate and vincristine for 2–3 cycles. If the disease continues to remain inoperable or progresses, the patient should receive preoperative RT, or in some case, RT alone. Pisansky et al. [14] compared once-daily radiation administered preoperatively at a dose of 50.4 Gy over 28 days in 16 patients with twice-daily radiation given preoperatively at a dose of 44.2 Gy over 13 days in 13 patients. Patients administered the twice-daily treatment appeared less likely to fail locally than patients treated with daily irradiation, with an 8 % local recurrence risk (RR) at 5 years and a median time to disease progression of 17 months in the twice-daily group versus 26 % and 13 months in the once-daily group.

Postoperative Radiotherapy

If inflammatory breast cancer is considered inoperable at presentation, it should be treated initially with neoadjuvant CT [15]. Patients should be carefully monitored for response, and after achieving maximal clinical response, patients should be reevaluated for mastectomy. About 80 % of patients with IBC will achieve clinical response, and their disease will become operable [16]. All patients should receive postmastectomy RT delivered to the chest wall and the lymph nodes [17].

Liauw et al. [18] reported their experience with 61 patients with IBC who were treated curatively from 1982 to 2001. Although postmastectomy RT was delivered utilizing once-daily fractionation schedules, the authors concluded that total radiation doses of >60 Gy resulted in better freedom from locoregional disease progression and that local control was strongly predictive of better cause-specific survival ($p=0.0003$). However, 22 % of the patients in this study developed locally recurrent disease as a component of failure. In an attempt to further decrease these local RR, the authors have now adopted the use of hyperfractionated RT for their patients with IBC [19].

Concurrent Radiotherapy

Despite the clear advantages of adjuvant chemoradiation strategies at other disease sites such as gynecological, gastrointestinal, and head and neck malignancies as extensively explored in breast cancer therapy [20], preliminary experience employing concurrent Xeloda and radiation in 55 patients with inoperable breast cancer has been favorable, with 91 % of these patients converting to operable. The clinical CR was 33 %; moreover, the overall pathological complete RR was 20 %. In general, patients have tolerated this treatment well with very few additional acute side effects, and as such, this may represent an alternative strategy to dose acceleration/escalation in patients with IBC at high risk for local failure.

Genet et al. [21] conducted a study between 1990 and 2000; 66 patients with nonmetastatic IBC were treated with CT and concomitant irradiation. Induction CT consisted of epirubicin, cyclophosphamide, and vindesine in association with split-course bifractionated irradiation at a total dose of 65 Gy with concomitant cisplatin and 5-fluorouracil. Median OS was 63 months, and median follow-up was 55.5 months.

Dose escalation in IBC is characterized by a high rate of locoregional recurrence after surgery alone and the rapid appearance of distant metastases. However, long-term survival is possible for patients presenting with this diagnosis and treated with multimodality therapy.

Due to poor LRC rates for this disease, dose escalation beyond the dose used to treat non-IBC appears warranted. Given the rarity of this disease, there have been, to our knowledge, no dose-escalation trials, but hyperfractionation has been reported to yield better local control rates compared with historical controls, and data from numerous other sites may be extrapolated to provide insight into safe means of escalating treatment for this aggressive disease [22]. Arguments may be made for dose escalation with standard fractionation, hyperfractionation, and/or concurrent CT. Integrating first principles regarding dose from other sites into standard treatment approaches for noninflammatory guidelines has guided the following approach with respect to dose in our experience and practice.

Accelerated Hyperfractionated Radiation

To offset the rapidly proliferative potential of IBC [23], researchers began investigating accelerated hyperfractionated RT. This strategy uses twice-daily treatments to shorten the treatment course and thereby minimize the risk of tumor repopulation during therapy.

Accelerated treatment might be defined as the same total dose delivered in one-half of the overall time by means of the expediency of administering two or more fractions each day. In practice, it is never possible to achieve this because the acute effects become limiting. It is necessary either to interpose a rest period in mid-treatment or to reduce the dose slightly with acute effects as the limiting factor. The intent of this accelerated treatment strategy is to reduce repopulation in a rapidly proliferating tumor. There should be little or no change in late effects because the number of fractions and doses-per-fraction are unaltered. Arthur et al. [24] report that after induction CT, RT was delivered using an accelerated superfractionated schedule; the majority of patients were treated utilizing 1.5-Gy fractions delivered twice daily with a 6-h interfraction interval. Total dose was 45 Gy over 3 weeks, and the bolus is used on the skin of the breast throughout the entire treatment, with a 20-Gy boost in ten fractions to the entire breast. Total radiation dose was 63–66 Gy delivered during 4–5 weeks. Therefore, modified radical mastectomy after accelerated superfractionated RT was reserved for patients with persistent or progressive disease. Five-year OS for complete responders was 68 %; this is in contrast to the 5-year OS rate of 14 % rate observed with incomplete responders. Five-year actuarial DFS and OS rates for the entire patient cohort were 11 and 33 %, respectively.

Patients with IBC who are able to complete treatment with CT, mastectomy, and postmastectomy radiation have a high probability of LRC. Bristol et al. [25] found that an excellent LRC rate was achieved with lower morbidity with a 60-Gy dose.

Escalation of the postmastectomy radiation dose to 66 Gy appears to benefit patients with disease that responds poorly to CT, those with positive, close, or unknown margin status and those aged <45 years. Liao et al. [3] reviewed the results of 115 patients with IBC and concluded that escalating the dose from 60 to 66 Gy delivered by twice-daily fractionation significantly improved the 5-year LRC rate (58 vs. 84 %, respectively; $p = 0.04$).

An aggressive locoregional treatment strategy, including RT to the chest wall and training lymph nodes to 51 Gy followed by a chest-wall boost dose to 66 Gy, may be justified for patients with poor response to neoadjuvant CT, those with positive or unknown surgical margin status and those <45 years of age.

Patients >45 year of age with good response to neoadjuvant CT receive a taxane along with their doxorubicin-based CT, with negative surgical margins, and with fewer than four evolved lymph nodes, can be treated at a lower total dose than 60 Gy.

Initial Staging Studies in Radiation Treatment Planning

Radiation therapy treatment planning and delivery capabilities have changed dramatically since the introduction of three-dimensional treatment planning and are continuing to change relatively rapidly in response to the implementation of new advanced technologies. Three-dimensional conformal radiation therapy (3DCRT) is now firmly in place as the standard of practice in clinics around the world.

Comprehensive pre-CT imaging with the specific goal of localizing gross disease in three dimensions for its targeting during radiation planning is critical for these patients. Because of the locally aggressive nature of this disease, pre-therapy images often illustrate the natural locoregional progression of breast cancer from the breast through the axillary lymph node levels into the supraclavicular (SC) fossa [26].

The aggressive but local nature of IBC leads to novel challenges for RT. The skin is clearly at higher risk for recurrence than in noninflammatory breast cancer (IBC), and common findings suspicion disease at presentation based on the presence of gross disease in the infraclavicular, SC, or internal mammary lymph node basins necessitate individualized targeting and conformal CT-based treatment planning. Response to treatment and extent of nodal resection must be taken into account in designing fields and choosing the treatment dose.

Positron emission tomography (PET)/computed tomography (CT) imaging detected new areas of disease that were not appreciated with conventional imaging and physical examination.

The information currenüy offered by PET-CT should be considerer for the initial standing In IBC patients. It appears that some prognostic information can be derived from 18-fluoro-deoxy-glucose (FDG) uptake characteristics.

PET/CT provides functional information localized to axial CT data, which can be later correlated to radiation-planning CT scans. PET/CT scans also generally include high neck imaging; thus, SC and cervical nodes can be fully visualized [27, 28]. Regional nodal ultrasound (US) is

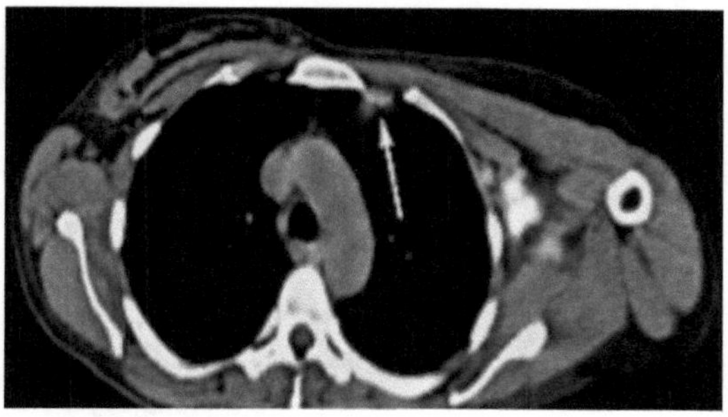

Fig. 7.1 18-Fluoro-deoxy-glucose *arrow* FDG avid internal mammary lymph node in a patient with IBC

an excellent modality in experienced hands to evaluate the regional nodes and biopsy when indicated; however, without additional CT-based localization, this information will generally require large radiation boost fields to unresected gross regional disease guided by anatomic boundaries (i.e., the SC fossa) rather than fields tailored to gross disease and appropriate clinical margins (Fig. 7.1).

However, PET/CT has limitations, there may be causes of false positives, and in our institution is not routinely used.

Conventional Simulation Technique

Simulation and Field Design

Patients are placed on a 10–15° angle board to flatten the chest-wall slope in the region of the sternum. CT simulation is preferred in order to optimize target definition (Fig. 7.3).

Postsurgical range-of-motion exercise is critical to allow the arm to rest comfortably and sufficiently high so that the border between the SC field and the tangents can be placed at the inferior border of the head of the clavicle. After raising the arm sufficiently to ensure that the soft tissue of the arm is out-of-field, the arm should not be overextended. This balance allows for minimal skin fold in the SC cervical junction to prevent desquamation in the shoulder region. The patient's head should be turned approximately 45° past midline toward the opposite side to allow access to the SC and cervical nodes. Under-rotation of the neck maintains the chin in the field, while over-rotation of the head will limit accessibility to the nodes and necessitate a large angle using an anterior-posterior oblique approach.

The treatment fields are designed to conform to the chest wall of each patient, potentially avoiding the lung tissue. This is accomplished by the use of an external marker on the chest wall that can be observed under fluoroscopy or on simulation film; the marker comprises a piece of soldering wire placed along the chest wall at midline and conforming to the chest-wall contour. Patients should be immobilized with their ipsilateral arm adduced and externally rotated. In assessing arm position, it is important to have access to the soft tissues.

Radiopaque Mark

Scars and drain sites should be marked with radiopaque mark wires to guide field design, and field borders may be marked with radiopaque mark wires as well. At this point, setup reproducibility may be improved by asking the patient to sit up and resettle into the immobilization device prior to scanning. This simulates the small differences in positioning within the cradle that will occur during treatment. Setup reproducibility is critical in the setting of locally advanced breast cancer (LABC), in which high-dose conformal boost fields may be required. CT images are subsequently acquired and employed for isocenter placement.

Setup and Field Arrangement

The modern techniques rely on CT-based treatment planning permit to establish the anatomy relationship to the chest wall, heart, and lung.

Acquisition of Planning CT Data

The patients are placed for CT scanning in the supine position with their arms above the head in

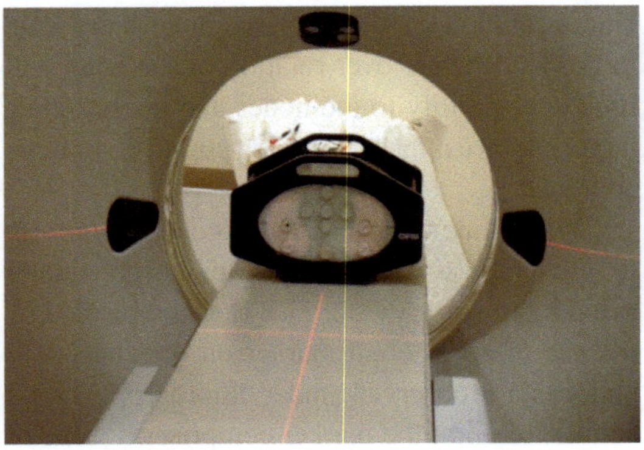

Fig. 7.2 CT simulator with phantom

arm support. The CT images were obtained at 3-mm slice thickness from the level of the mandible down to the diaphragm.

CT-Based Treatment Planning

The use of a CT simulator and virtual simulation is preferable for treatment planning purposes in that the latter permit 3D visualization of targets and normal tissues. A fluoroscopic simulator can be used to set up the treatment for the chest wall and regional nodes if CT technology is not available. In either case, the chest-wall field borders should be clinically determined and tentatively delineated by the radiation oncologist (Fig. 7.2).

While it is generally feasible to treat breast cancer utilizing fluoroscopic-based radiation treatment planning, the high likelihood of regional gross disease in IBC and the expected toxicity from aggressive RT approaches render CT-based treatment planning the preferred approach for superior coverage and dose homogeneity. Contouring gross disease and clinical target volumes is extremely helpful in dose prescription so that the entire volume at risk is covered and can be fully assessed. Incorporating additional fields to improve conformality and dose homogeneity can allow for full coverage of target volumes with appropriate dose without risking significant hot spots above critical structures [28] (Fig. 7.3).

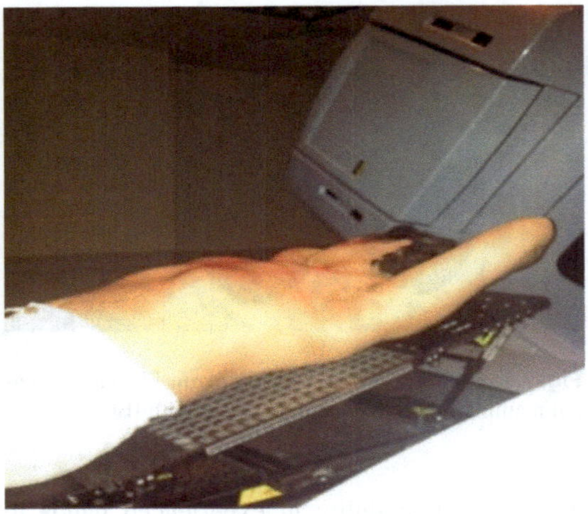

Fig. 7.3 After mastectomy being treated with radiotherapy in our institution

Technique

There not exists a consensus above the best technique for IBC; however, several techniques are available to treat the supraclavicular region, chest wall, and internal mammary lymph nodes [29–31]. Kuske et al. [29] have proposed a technique with 5-field for the comprehensive coverage of the chest wall, internal mammary, axillary, and supraclavicular lymphatics for IBC (Fig. 7.4).

One of the more common methods is to utilize a 15–25° oblique electron field to treat the lateral border of IM. This is then matched to a pair of photon tangent fields that treat the lateral chest wall and that are created with matched non-divergent deep and cranial borders. A couch and non-divergent deep border is achieved by over-rotating the gantry or a half-beam block. The collimators are rotated to match the chest-wall slope, and any volume that extends into the SC field is blocked. An alternative technique that is of particular benefit for patients with very little tissue between the lung and the skin is to use three-electron fields. Regardless of the technique employed, it is important to avoid high doses of radiation to the heart when considering different treatment techniques for left-sided lesions. In a comparison of heart doses utilizing several postmastectomy chest-wall techniques, Pierce et al. [32] noted that the volume

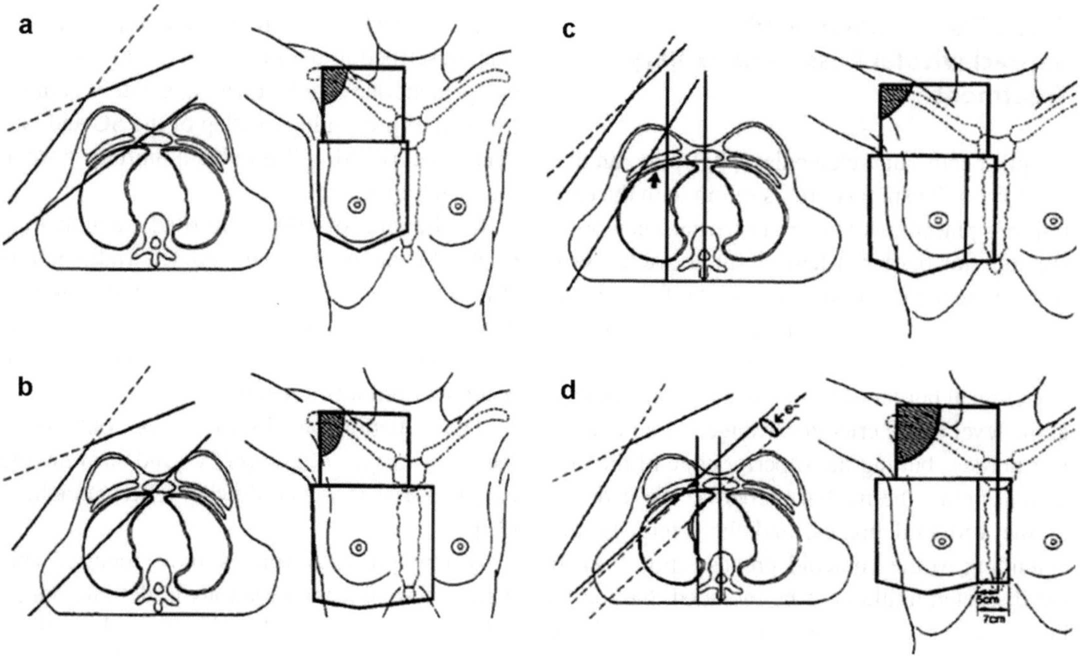

Fig. 7.4 (**a**) The standard tangential/supraclavicular three-field technique does not include internal mammary IM. (**b**) Broad tangents can irradiate an excessive volume of lung. (**c**) Cool triangle (*arrow*) between the tangential field and an anterior internal mammary port is more dramatic with an intact breast than a chest wall after mastectomy. (**d**) The five-field technique for comprehensive chest wall/nodal irradiation

of the heart receiving ≥30 Gy was least extensive using partially wide tangent fields and, as expected, greatest when using cobalt techniques.

A multi-isocenter technique is used to avoid limiting the tangent field to one-half of the maximum, as occurs when employing a mono-isocentric technique and treating the tangents with a half-beam block. Although either approach works for the majority of patients, field margins are routinely larger for patients with IBC. The medial chest wall is treated with an electron field prescribed to cover the internal mammary lymph nodes in the first three interspaces with the 90 % isodose line. This necessitates a steeper tangent angle, providing greater coverage of the chest wall's posterior lateral border. The remainder of the chest wall is treated with standard photon tangent fields, and the tangent and internal mammary fields are matched on the skin. This approach minimizes the volume of lung treated and excludes the heart entirely from the tangent fields. Because the medial internal mammary field extends the length of the tangent field and is used to treat the medial portion of the chest wall, the heart may receive a significant dose from the internal mammary field when high-energy electrons are required to cover the internal mammary in the first three interspaces. In this case, the internal mammary can be split into two fields, choosing more superficial electron energy in the lower field to eliminate the heart from the high-dose region.

Increasing the couch angle generates a non-divergent superior border between the tangents and the SC field, and rotating the gantry creates a non-divergent deep border. The SC field is treated with a half-beam block. To intensify the dose to the skin, a 3-mm tissue equivalent bolus is employed over the chest wall and infraclavicular fossa with the goal of developing brisk erythema throughout these regions by the end of treatment. In addition, all adjacent field edges are overlapped by 3 mm either in treatment planning or clinically at the time of treatment each day to ensure adequate coverage of these junctions.

Three-Field Technique of Supraclavicular Fossa and Axillary Treatment

A split-beam supraclavicular (SC) port, angled 15–20° off the spinal cord, is set up with the central axis placed just above the sternal-manubrial, the superior border at least 2 cm above the skin flash at the top of the supraclavicular fossa, junction can be matched to the chest-wall fields to target the SC fossa and axillary apex. The superior clinical border of this field is typically placed at the level of the cricoid cartilage, with the inferior border abutting the superior edge of the tangential fields, the medial border on the pedicles of the vertebral bodies, and the lateral border extending to the coracoid process (Fig. 7.4). If the dissected axilla is to be included, the lateral border of the SC field is extended to the middle axilla.

The geometric edges of the SC inferior border and superior border of the tangential fields must be aligned in order for there to be no divergence of the three beams, which would cause hot spots and overdosing in the overlap regions. Several techniques have been described to match these fields, all of which are effective in producing a uniform dose across the match line. This technique requires that the clinical borders be tentatively determined and that the isocenter location be determined along the match line of the SC and tangent fields in the superior to inferior, anterior to posterior, and medial to lateral axis either during fluoroscopic or CT (virtual) simulation (Fig. 7.5). During treatment, the three fields are treated in succession without movement of the isocenter. Although blocks can be used (i.e., to block the lung or heart in the tangential fields or the spinal cord and central structures in the SC field), no blocks are required with this technique to achieve matching between the tangents and the SC field (Fig. 7.6).

Another commonly utilized technique is the rod-and-chain [33]; this method utilizes tabletop rotation, gantry and collimator angles, and corner blocks to match the SC field to the tangents and is not limited by the 20-cm tangent field size. Several other matching techniques employing different blocking methods [29, 32] have also been described in the literature. All of the previously mentioned techniques adequately achieve the goal of preventing overlap of the SC and tangential fields and will provide a uniform dose at the match line.

In the era of 3D conformal radiotherapy (3DCRT), an intensity-modulated radiotherapy (IMRT), accurate delineation of tumor volumes and surrounding normal structures becomes the most important task for subsequent treatment planning optimization and delivery.

The radiation oncologist draws contours of the gross target volume (GTV) and surrounding organs-at-risk (OAR) following ICRU guidelines [34].

A few previous studies have reported that there are significant variations in defining target volumes for breast RT [35]. To reduce these inconsistencies, the European Society of Therapeutic Radiology and Oncology (ESTRO) and Radiation Therapy Oncology Group (RTOG) initiated several independent studies for creating consensus guidelines for delineation of tumor volumes and surrounding OAR.

Use of Bolus

To intensify the dose to the skin, a 3-mm tissue equivalent bolus is used over the chest wall and infraclavicular fossa with the goal of developing brisk erythema throughout these regions by the end of treatment. Excellent locoregional control was observed in the population with IBC, patients who received standard fractionation radiation with daily skin bolus and taxanes as part of combined-modality therapy.

Damast et al. [36] reported that patients received chemotherapy (95 % anthracycline and 95 % taxane), modified radical mastectomy, and RT to the chest wall and regional lymph nodes using standard fractionation to 50 Gy and daily skin bolus. RT to the chest wall was delivered via electrons (55 %) or photons (45 %) in daily fractions of 180 cGy (73 %) or 200 cGy (27 %). Scar boost was performed in 11 %. A majority (84 %) of patients completed the prescribed treatment.

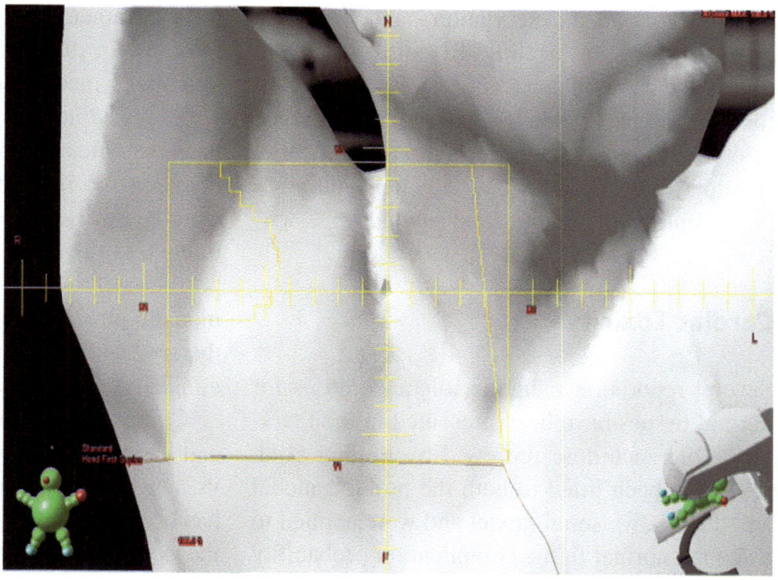

Fig. 7.5 Supraclavicular (*SC*) fossa and axillary treatment

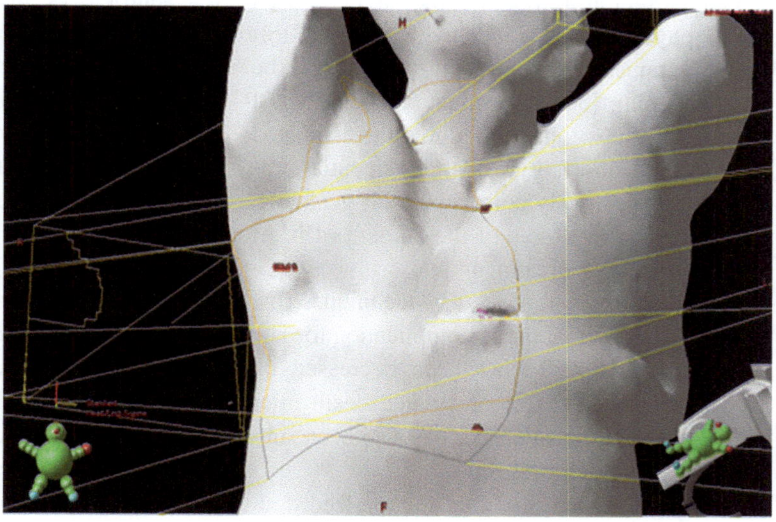

Fig. 7.6 3D planning. Axillo-supraclavicular and tangential fields. Three-dimensional conformal treatment planning in the patient in the tomography

Median follow-up was 47 months (range, 10–134 months). Locoregional control (LRC) at 3 and at 5 years was 90 and 87 %, respectively.

Toxicity

Acute Toxicity

Aggressive management of acute toxicity is critical to completing any aggressive radiation schedule without a treatment break. Examination of the impact of treatment duration on local control in breast cancer and other sites has clearly demonstrated a direct relationship between treatment delays and protracted treatment courses and local failure. Both patient and radiation oncologist need to be prepared for significant moist desquamation toward the end of treatment, particularly in patients with large body habitus in whom eliminating skin folds through treatment setup is not entirely possible. Early treatments with protective, chemical-free emollients to provide moisture are beneficial. Topical gel applications can prevent continued excoriation and infection, thereby promoting healing of moist desquamation. Patients should be assured that acute skin toxicity will heal but that it will progress at home prior to resolution, and appropriate pain relief should be prescribed to support patients throughout completion of therapy and beyond.

Cardiac Toxicity

Several reports on radiation tolerance doses for normal tissues have been presented in the literature. Tolerance dose proposed by Emami et al. [37] have been fitted to both the prohibit model and the relative serial model and were applied to calculate normal tissue complication probability predictions (NTCP).

Gagliardi et al. [38] and Hurkman et al. used one biophysical NTCP model with one set of tolerance parameters for each the two ORAs, the heart and lung [39], to evaluate various breast irradiation setups. They found that the estimated excess cardiac mortality risk after tangential irradiation was positively correlated with geometrical/anatomical measures of the amount of heart included inside the treatment fields.

With the use of modern-day techniques, the probability of normal tissue complication for late cardiac tissue toxicity has been decreased by 30–50 % [40]. The risk of cardiac death after adjuvant RT for breast cancer has also been substantially decreased over time.

Several meta-analyses of the randomized studies of the first-generation postmastectomy therapy trials have suggested that the benefit of radiation, with respect to survival, was counteracted by cardiac mortality, which appeared to be related with vascular/coronary-associated deaths from unintended radiation of the coronary and carotid arteries [41]. When analyzed further, these findings of cardiac deaths were significantly more apparent in older trials from Europe [41–43], which used outdated techniques and equipment (i.e., en face chest-wall photon fields, cobalt-60 units, larger fractionation size). Further supporting this observation, the risk of cardiac mortality has shown to be significantly higher in patients with radiation for left- rather than for right-sided breast cancers [44, 45]. In different studies that compared the treatments made available in units of cobalt-60 with megavoltage units, doses to the heart have been significantly reduced; no difference was noted in the incidence of mortality from ischemic heart disease between left- and right-sided tumors. Furthermore, data from the most modern postmastectomy trials suggest that combined-modality treatment with mastectomy, systemic therapy, and adjuvant radiation did not result in clinically relevant cardiotoxic effects.

Comparison of the volume of heart irradiated and the dose received for the standard tangential vs. newer, more conformal radiation techniques has been difficult to evaluate for several reasons: the definition of the organ-at-risk has not been well defined or consistent (i.e., whole heart vs. left ventricle vs. myocardium); dosimetric data for historic techniques have not been well reported, and clinical manifestations of cardiac toxicity often occur with a latency period of >10 years after treatment with endpoints that are often difficult to measure (i.e., pericarditis, coronary artery disease leading to angina, myocardial infarction, and thromboemboli), with no established surrogates for clinical toxicity (i.e., perfusion studies) other than death from cardiac causes. Based on the guidelines in the Radiation Therapy Oncology Group (RTOG) Breast Cancer Atlas Project, the entire heart should be contoured. Cardiac doses should be measured to generate a dose-volume histogram (DVH) to allow for accurate assessment of the dose to several portions of the heart [46].

Three-dimensional planning with CT-generated contours can be more precisely customized to the individual patient with analysis of the dose volumes for critical structures.

Several modern maneuvers for chest-wall radiation have been shown to reduce the volume of the heart irradiated. Breath-holding techniques (using active or unassisted breathing control devices) and respiratory gating have been shown as effective techniques to reduce cardiac volumes [47–49]; in addition, advancements in patient treatment positioning have made a significant difference in the amount of heart irradiated.

There are several treatment-related factors that have shown to increase cardiac toxicity, including intentional treatment of the lower IM nodes. When the lower IM nodes are intentionally included in chest-wall radiation, the volume of heart irradiated has been shown to increase, particularly when an additional IM field is added [50]. When adding a separate IM field, it is prudent to use a combination of electrons and photons or electrons alone (as opposed to an en face photon field) and to obtain a treatment plan in which cardiac doses are minimized.

Radiation Pneumonitis

Symptomatic radiation pneumonitis is uncommon when only the breast is irradiated following breast-conserving therapy. It typically onsets 2–3 months after completing treatment with a clinical syndrome of cough, fever, shortness of breath, and radiologic changes confined to the radiation therapy field. Symptoms can persist for several weeks and in general are self-limiting. Pulmonary fibrosis typically follows in the affected portion of the lung [51].

The incidence of pulmonary toxicity after RT for breast cancer varies significantly in the literature but is typically well under 10 % with modern treatment units and techniques. Although the majority of studies assessing radiation-induced pneumonitis have been performed in patients after breast-conservation therapy and not specifically in the postmastectomy setting, acute and long-term effects are similar in that they are primarily dependent on the volume of lung irradiated, thus higher with the addition of SC or IM fields. Furthermore, the use and sequencing of systemic therapy clearly impact the rate of pneumonitis, with a significantly higher risk when concurrent vs. sequential RT is delivered [52].

Although the ultimate incidence-of-pulmonary-toxicity endpoint differs significantly based on the method used to quantify pulmonary complications, whether it be patients' symptom assessment, chest x-rays, pulmonary function testing, perfusion studies, or CT scans, several studies have suggested that the frequency of pulmonary toxicity can be predicted based on the amount of lung in the tangential fields [53]. Although several models for predicting lung toxicity after breast RT have been proposed in the literature, no specific model has been consistently utilized in clinical practice or in the literature.

Lymphedema

After treatment, upper-extremity arm edema is a commonly experienced complication. Similar to issues regarding lung toxicity measurements, the frequency of lymphedema is variable depending on the definition used, whether it is patient vs. lymphedema specialist assessment or subjective severity vs. quantitative measurements. The risk of lymphedema increases with the extent of lymph nodes excised and is higher after RT is administered to the dissected axilla [54].

Other known risk factors include more advanced age and obesity (high body mass index [BMI]). There is some data suggesting that the addition of an SC field to tangential fields and the use of a posterior axillary boost field may increase the risk of lymphedema in node-positive patients.

Brachial Plexopathy

Brachial plexopathy after radiation therapy is uncommon and typically seen only when regional nodal irradiation has been delivered. The clinical syndrome most frequently presents with paresthesias and is associated with pain and/or weakness in the ipsilateral arm.

The mechanism of radiation-induced brachial plexopathy is not completely understood, but it is suspected that fibrosis of tissue around peripheral nerves occurs with injury to small vessels that leads to ischemia. Pathologic studies have shown loss of myelin, fibrosis and thickening of the neurolemma sheath, and obliteration of the vasonevum.

Because the brachial plexus transverses the SC field into the axilla, it needs to be considered an organ-at-risk with the potential for significant toxicity. The effects of dose, volume, and fractionation need to be well thought through, just as with the remaining organs-at-risk. Long-term sequelae of radiation to the brachial plexus include radiation-induced brachial plexopathy, a clinical syndrome in which patients who have had previous SC fossa/axillary radiation present symptoms of arm numbness, tingling, pain, or motor weakness months to years after treatment. When these symptoms occur, a workup to rule out neoplastic infiltration of tumor recurrence is imperative [55].

To ensure minimizing the risk of radiation-induced brachial plexopathy, it is important to perform the following: (1) significantly reduce hot spots in the supraclavicular/axillary field (SAF), (2) avoid the use of large doses per fraction, and (3) place the match line for the SAF below the level of the brachial plexus whenever possible.

Conclusions

In conclusion, combined-modality therapy using doxorubicin-based chemotherapy, mastectomy, and postmastectomy radiation provides excellent LRC and reasonable 5-year survival rates for patients with IBC who successfully complete the planned treatment course. Aggressive locoregional treatment strategies including hyperfractionated radiation therapy to the chest wall and draining lymph nodes at 51 Gy followed by a chest-wall boost dose at 66 Gy may be justified for patients with high-risk features. Concurrent chemoradiation strategies should be considered and explored in patients at high risk for this disease. Highly selected patients with CR to neoadjuvant CT, with negative surgical margins, with four or more lymph nodes involved, and who are treated with taxane-based CT in addition to doxorubicin-based CT can be treated with a total dose <60 Gy. The advances made in imaging-based radiation treatment planning clearly play a role in the management and design of RT in IBC and should be fully used to tailor treatment fields based on localization of initially gross disease, response to CT, and extent of dissection. Multidisciplinary collaboration and management are critical in ensuring optimal treatment.

References

1. Bristol IJ, et al. Inflammatory breast cancer: current concepts in local management. Breast Dis. 2005;22:75–83.
2. Harris EE, et al. Ten-year outcome after combined modality therapy for inflammatory breast cancer. Int J Radiat Oncol Biol Phys. 2003;55(5):1200–8.
3. Liao Z, et al. Locoregional irradiation for inflammatory breast cancer: effectiveness of dose escalation in decreasing recurrence. Int J Radiat Oncol Biol Phys. 2000;47(5):1191–200.
4. Fleming RY, Asmar L, Buzdar AU, et al. Effectiveness of mastectomy by response to induction chemotherapy for control in inflammatory breast carcinoma. Ann Surg Oncol. 1997;4:452–61.
5. Barker JL, Nelson AJ, Montague ED. Inflammatory carcinoma of the breast. Radiology. 1976;121:173–6.
6. Panades M, Olivotto IA, Speers CH, et al. Evolving treatment strategies for inflammatory breast cancer: a population-based survival analysis. J Clin Oncol. 2005;23(9):1941–50.
7. Ueno NT, Buzdar AU, Singletary SE, Ames FC, McNeese MD, Holmes FA, et al. Combined-modality treatment of inflammatory breast carcinoma: twenty years of experience at M.D. Anderson Cancer Center. Cancer Chemother Pharmacol. 1997;40(4):321–9.
8. Rousse J, Friedman S, Sarrazin D, et al. Primary chemotherapy in treatment of inflammatory breast carcinoma: a study of 230 cases for the Institut Gustave-Roussy. J Clin Oncol. 1986;4:1765–71.
9. Thoms Jr WW, et al. Multimodal treatment for inflammatory breast cancer. Int J Radiat Oncol Biol Phys. 1998;17:739–45.
10. Mourali N, Tabbane F, Muenz LR, Behi J, Ben Moussa F, Jaziri M, et al. Ten-year results utilizing chemotherapy as primary treatment in nonmetastatic, rapidly progressing breast cancer. Cancer Invest. 1993;11(4):363–70.
11. De Boer RH, Allum WH, Ebbs S, et al. Multimodality therapy in inflammatory breast cancer: is there a place for surgery? Ann Oncol. 2000;11:1147–53.
12. Fleming RY. Effectiveness of mastectomy by response to induction chemotherapy for control in inflammatory breast carcinoma. Ann Surg Oncol. 1997;4(6):452–61.
13. Dawood S, Cristofanilli M. Oncology inflammatory breast cancer: what progress have we made? Oncology (Williston Park). 2011;25(3):264–70.
14. Pisansky TM, et al. Inflammatory breast cancer: integration of irradiation, surgery, and chemotherapy. Am J Clin Oncol. 1992;15(5):376–87.

15. Chu AM, Wood WC, Doucette JA. Inflammatory breast carcinoma treated by radical radiotherapy. Cancer. 1980;45:2730–7.
16. Pérez CA, Fields JN, Fracasso PM, et al. Management of locally advanced carcinoma of the breast. II: inflammatory carcinoma. Cancer. 1994;74(1 Suppl): 466–76.
17. Rouesse J, Friedman S, Sarrazin D, et al. Primary chemotherapy in the treatment of inflammatory breast carcinoma: a study of 230 cases for the Institut Gustave-Roussy. J Clin Oncol. 1986;4:1765–71.
18. Liauw SL, et al. Inflammatory breast carcinoma: outcomes with trimodality therapy for nonmetastatic disease. Cancer. 2004;100(5):920–8.
19. Thames Jr HD, et al. Accelerated fractionation vs. hyperfractionation: rationales for several treatments per day. Int J Radiat Oncol Biol Phys. 1983;9(2): 127–38.
20. Cox JD. Chemoradiation for malignant epithelial tumors. Cancer Radiother. 1998;2(1):7–11.
21. Genet D, et al. Concomitant intensive chemoradiotherapy induction in non-metastatic inflammatory breast cancer: long-term follow-up. Br J Cancer. 2007;97(7):883–7.
22. Hasbini A, Le Pechoux C, Roche B, et al. Alternating chemotherapy and hyperfractionated accelerated radiotherapy in non-metatastic inflammatory breast cancer. Cancer Radiother. 2000;4:265–73.
23. Barker JL, Montague ED, et al. Clinical experience with irradiation of inflammatory carcinoma of the breast with and without elective chemotherapy. Cancer. 1980;45:625–9.
24. Arthur DW, et al. Accelerated superfractionated radiotherapy for inflammatory breast carcinoma: complete response predicts outcome and allows for breast conservation. Int J Radiat Oncol Biol Phys. 1999;44(2): 289–96.
25. Bristol IJ, et al. Locoregional treatment outcomes after multimodality management of inflammatory breast cancer. Int J Radiat Oncol Biol Phys. 2008; 72(2):474–84.
26. Woodward WA, et al. The role of locoregional therapy in inflammatory breast cancer. Semin Oncol. 2008; 35(1):78–86.
27. Walker GV, et al. Pretreatment staging positron emission tomography/computed tomography inpatients with inflammatory breast cancer influences radiation treatment field designs. Int J Radiat Oncol Biol Phys. 2012;8(1):1381–86.
28. Alberini JL, et al. 18F-fluorodeoxyglucose positron emission tomography/computed tomography (FDG-PET/CT) imaging in the staging and prognosis of inflammatory breast cancer. Cancer. 2009;115(21): 5038–47.
29. Kuske RR, et al. Diagnosis and management of inflammatory breast cancer. Sem Radiat Oncol. 1994;4:270–82.
30. Marks LB, et al. To treat or not to treat the internal mammary nodes. Int J Radiat Oncol Biol Phys. 1994;29:903–9.
31. Siddon SL, et al. Three-field technique for breast irradiation using tangential field corner blocks. Int J Radiat Oncol Biol Phys. 1983;9:583–8.
32. Pierce LJ, et al. Postmastectomy radiotherapy of the chest wall: dosimetric comparison of common techniques. Int J Radiat Oncol Biol Phys. 2002;52(5): 1220–30.
33. Chu JC, Solin LJ, Hwang CC, et al. A non-divergent three field matching technique for breast irradiation. Int J Radiat Oncol Biol Phys. 1990;19:1037–40.
34. International Commission on Radiation Units and Measurements (ICRU). Prescribing, recording and reporting photon beam therapy (supplement to ICRU report 50), Bethesda, 1999.
35. Landis DM, Luo W, Son J, et al. Variability among breast radiation oncologist in delineation of postsurgical lumpectomy cavity. Int J Radiat Oncol Biol Phys. 2007;67:1299–308.
36. Damast S, et al. Locoregional outcomes of inflammatory breast cancer patients treated with standard fractionation radiation and daily skin bolus in the taxane era. Int J Radiat Oncol Biol Phys. 2010;77(4): 1105–12.
37. Emamin B, Lyman J, Brown A, et al. Tolerance of normal tissue to therapeutic irradiation. Int J Radiat Oncol Biol Phys. 1991;21:109–22.
38. Gagliardi G, Lax I, Rutqvist LE. Partial irradiation of the heart. Semin Radiat Oncol. 2000;11:224–5.
39. Hurkmans CW, Borger JH, et al. Cardiac and lung complication probabilities after breast cancer irradiation. Radiother Oncol. 2000;55:145–51.
40. Muren LP, Maurstad G, Hafslund R, et al. Cardiac and pulmonary doses and complication probabilities in standard and conformal tangential irradiation in conservative management of breast cancer. Radiother Oncol. 2002;62:173–83.
41. Jones J, Ribeiro G. Mortality patterns over 34 years of breast cancer patients in a clinical trial of post-operative radiotherapy. Clin Radiol. 1989;40:204–8.
42. Haybittle JL, Brinkley D, Houghton J, et al. Postoperative radiotherapy and late mortality: evidence from the cancer research campaign trial for early breast cancer. BMJ. 1989;298:1611–4.
43. Fuller SA, Haybittle JL, Smith RE, et al. Cardiac doses in post-operative breast irradiation. Radiother Oncol. 1992;25:19–24.
44. Hurkmans CW, Cho BC, Damen E, et al. Reduction of cardiac and lung complication probabilities after breast irradiation using conformal radiotherapy with or without intensity modulation. Radiother Oncol. 2002;62:163–71.
45. Hojris I, Overgaard M, Christensen JJ, et al. Morbidity and mortality of ischemic heart disease in high-risk breast-cancer patients after adjuvant postmastectomy systemic treatment with or without radiotherapy: analysis of DBCG 82b and 82c randomized trials. Lancet. 1999;354:1425–30.
46. Moran MS, Haffty BG. Radiation techniques and toxicities for local advanced breast cancer. Semin Radiat Oncol. 2009;19:244–55. Lu HM, Cash E, Chen MH,

et al. Reduction of cardiac volume in left-breast treatment fields by respiratory maneuvers: a CT study. Int J Radiat Oncol Biol Phys. 2000;47:895–904.
47. Korreman SS, Pedersen AN, Nottrup TJ, et al. Breathing adapted radiotherapy for breast cancer: comparison of free breathing gating with the breath-hold technique. Radiother Oncol. 2005;76:311–8.
48. Remouchamps VM, Vicini FA, Sharpe MB, et al. Significant reductions in heart and lung doses using deep inspiration breath hold with active breathing control and intensity-modulated radiation therapy for patients treated with locoregional breast irradiation. Int J Radiat Oncol Biol Phys. 2003;55:392–406.
49. Canney PA, Deehan C, Glegg M, et al. Reducing cardiac dose in post-operative irradiation of breast cancer patients: the relative importance of patient positioning and CT scan planning. Br J Radiol. 1999;72:986–93.
50. Gyenes G, Gagliardi G, Lax I, et al. Evaluation of irradiated heart volumes in stage I breast cancer patients treated with postoperative adjuvant radiotherapy. J Clin Oncol. 1997;15:1348–53.
51. Kimsey FC, Mendenhall NP, Ewald LM, et al. Is radiation treatment volume a predictor for acute or late effects on pulmonary function? A prospective study of patients treated with breast-conserving surgery and post-operative irradiation. Cancer. 1994;73:2549–55.
52. Lind P, Wennberg B, Gagliardi G, et al. Pulmonary complications following different radiotherapy techniques for breast cancer, and the association to irradiated lung volume and dose. Breast Cancer Res Treat. 2001;68:199–210.
53. Krengli M, Sacco M, Loi G, et al. Pulmonary changes after radiotherapy for conservative treatment of breast cancer: a prospective study. Int J Radiat Oncol Biol Phys. 2008;70:1460–7.
54. Svensson H, Westling P, Larsson L-G. Radiation-induced lesions of the brachial plexus correlated to the dose-time-fractionation schedule. Acta Radiol Ther Phys Biol. 1975;14:228–38.
55. Rubin D, Schomberg P, Shepard R, et al. Arteritis and brachial plexus neuropathy as delayed complications of radiation therapy. Mayo Clin Proc. 2001;76(8):849–52.

8 Recurrent Inflammatory Breast Carcinoma: Prevalence, Patterns of Recurrence, and Therapeutic Approach

Juan Alberto Serrano-Olvera, Claudia Arce-Salinas, David F. Cantu-de Leon, Luis Alonso Herrera-Montalvo, and Jaime G. de la Garza-Salazar

Introduction

Breast cancer represents the second most frequently found neoplasm among feminine population; at the worldwide level, during the year 2008, 1,380,000 new cases were registered, with predominance in developed countries. It represented the fifth cause of cancer-related deaths and induced 485,000 deaths during this time lapse [1]. An infrequent and aggressive of presentation of breast cancer is inflammatory carcinoma (IC), characterized by rapid growth, erythematous coloration of the skin (*peu d'orange*), and the majority of times, palpable mammary mass. In this mammary carcinoma variant, cutaneous biopsy of the histopathological study is peculiar; however, the basis of the diagnosis comprises the physical examination and the clinical history [2–4].

The incidence of inflammatory breast carcinoma (IBC) has not been precisely defined; notwithstanding this, it has been informed to range from 1 to 6 % [4, 5]. Apparently, among countries with less economic development and limitations in access to health systems, its incidence is greater; for example, it has been reported in Africa that IBC represents 68 % of cases with breast cancer [6], while in the USA, it only represents 1–2 %. For other countries, the frequency is variable (2.9 % Spain, 5.4 % France, 12 % Pakistan, 17.5 % in Nigeria, and up to 50 % in Tunisia). In the USA, between 1988 and 2000, an increase of 25 % among African-American women and of 19 % in Caucasian women was registered [3].

IBC is a particularly aggressive variant, with poor prognosis; its aggressivity can be due to its presentation in young women, with high-grade tumor histology and the absence of the expression of estrogen receptors [5]. Additionally, this disease is related with larger-sized neoplasms and with malignant cell-positive axillary lymph nodes [7]. Median survival among women affected by IC is limited to 3–4 years, but the survival expectancy can be less depending on the state of the hormonal receptors [7].

J.A. Serrano-Olvera, M.D. (✉)
Department of Clinical Research,
Instituto Nacional de Cancerologia-Mexico,
Ave. San Fernando # 22, Tlalpan, Mexico City,
DF 14080, Mexico
e-mail: serranoolvera@yahoo.com.mx

C. Arce-Salinas, M.D., M.Sc.
Department of Breast Tumor,
Instituto Nacional de Cancerologia-Mexico,
Mexico City, DF, Mexico

D.F. Cantu-de Leon, Ph.D.
Department of Clinical Research,
Instituto Nacional de Cancerologia-Mexico,
Ave. San Fernando # 22, Tlalpan, Mexico City,
DF 14080, Mexico

L.A. Herrera-Montalvo, Ph.D.
Department of Biomedic Research in Cancer,
Instituto Nacional de Cancerologia Mexico,
Mexico City, DF, Mexico

J.G. de la Garza-Salazar, M.D.
Department of Clinical Investigation,
Instituto Nacional de Cancerologia-Mexico,
Mexico City, DF, Mexico

J.G. de la Garza-Salazar et al. (eds.), *Inflammatory Breast Cancer*,
DOI 10.1007/978-0-85729-991-8_8, © Springer-Verlag London 2013

IBC always represents an advanced disease form. American Joint Committee on Cancer-Tumor-Node-Metastasis (AJCC-TNM) criteria classifies this presentation form as T4d. In the absence of proven lymph-node affectation, it can be considered as stage IIIB; with involvement of internal mammary-chain and supraclavicular lymph nodes (N3), it should be considered as stage IIIC, while the presence of distant metastasis qualifies the disease as stage IV [8, 9]. Seventy percent of cases are diagnosed in their locally advanced stage; thus, they are treated with the multimodal sequence integrated by neoadjuvant chemotherapy (CT), surgery, radiotherapy (RT), and/or endocrine therapy and/or biological therapy. However, a high proportion of patients experience disease recurrence. The purpose of this chapter is to evaluate the clinical behavior of recurrence and its current treatment options.

IBC: Is It Always an Advanced Disease?

At present, it is recognized that 70 % of cases of IBC are detected at a locally advanced disease stage (IIIB or IIIC) and that the remaining 30 % are classified with stage IV at the time of diagnosis; however, it is possible to consider that the proportion of stage IV could be >30 % from data deriving from diverse series. Brooks et al. [10], among 25 cases analyzed, detected metastatic disease in 68 %; Galmarini et al. [11], in 26 patients, observed 69 % in stage IIIB and 31 % in stage IV. Two reports with larger populations have been published; the Mayo Clinic (Rochester, MN, USA) reported that 17.9 % of 156 cases were classified at stage IV and the remainder, at stage IIIB [12], while the Canadian series found 92/485 cases (19 %) with M1 further than the supraclavicular lymph nodes [13].

Scarce prospective studies have been conducted to determine clinical-stage frequency in IBC; Mvere et al. [14] carried out a study to determine the frequency and metastatic pattern in women affected by locally advanced breast cancer (LABC) (inflammatory and noninflammatory); initial staging was performed by computed axial tomography. Thirty-eight (38 %) women were included in the group with IC and 59 (61 %) in the noninflammatory group; metastases at diagnosis were detected in 26 % of the first group and in 10 % of the second. However, depending on the method employed for analyzing the presence of distant disease, the prevalence of stage IV can vary. Carkaci et al. [15], among 41 women who were submitted to positron emission tomography-CT (PET/CT), 20 (49 %) showed distant hyper-uptake zones; of the latter, 11 (27 %) were localized at multiple sites and nine (22 %), at a sole site.

Standard Treatment for Inflammatory Breast Carcinoma

The multimodal therapy recognized as the standard primary treatment for women with IBC includes anthracyclines and/or taxanes during at least 6 cycles, followed by modified radical mastectomy and axillary lymph-node dissection without immediate reconstruction, radiotherapy (RT) that includes the chest wall and internal mammary and superclavicular lymph nodes, biological therapy with the monoclonal antibody trastuzumab in cases of overexpression of human epithelial growth factor receptor-2 (HER2), and adjuvant hormonotherapy for those with positive hormone-receptor expression [2, 8, 16].

Multimodal therapy has allowed increasing the expectancy of disease-free survival (DFS) in up to 40 versus 24 % with RT and surgery and in 6 % with only RT or surgery without CT [17]. However, aside from the planned and controlled studies, the proportion of cases that are in reality treated with the three therapeutic modalities is not 100 %; in addition, the order and sequence of treatments do not always result in being the same. Review of six series shows that between 76.7 and 100 % of cases receive primary CT [6, 18–22], mastectomy in 52–96 % [6, 18–21], and RT in 83–100 % [6, 18, 20, 21]. Notwithstanding this, one series that included 156 cases at the end of 1999 registered that only 65.8 % were treated with the combination of the three treatment forms [12], while, in more recent years, a small series identified the employment of trimodal therapy in 91 % of cases [22].

After the decade of the 1980s, the anthracyclines, and especially doxorubicin, have been the

Table 8.1 Results of the efficacy of neoadjuvant chemotherapy in inflammatory breast cancer

	N	Chemotherapy	ORR (%)	cCR (%)	pCR (%)	RFS or DFP	Survival
Labidi et al. [6]	93	Anthracycline	50	10	20	38 % at 3 years, TTP: 15 months	44 % at 3 years
Panades et al. [13]	148	Anthracycline/	NR	NR	28.4	NR	
	90	taxane	73.2	NR	NR	55.3 %	
Cristofanilli et al. [25]	178	Anthracycline	74	NR	10	26 months	41 months
	62	Anthracycline/ taxane	82	NR	25	31 months	52 months
Baldini et al. [19]	68	Anthracycline	73.6	NR	6	29 %	44 %
Ueno et al. [23]	172	Anthracycline	74	12	NR	44 % at 15 years with CR	51 % with CR
						31 % at 15 years with PR	31 % with PR
						7 % at 15 years with<PR	7 % with<PR
Harris et al. [21]	54	CMF or anthracycline	NR	73	12	34 % at 10 years	35 % at 10 years

N number of patients, *ORR* objective response rate, *cCR* complete clinical response, *pCR* pathological complete response, *RFS* recurrence-free survival, *PFS* progression-free survival, *TTP* time to progression, *NR* not reported, *CR* complete response, *PR* partial response

gold standard of neoadjuvant CT schemes for the treatment of IBC [12, 21]. Studies with the largest number of cases analyzed have utilized anthracycline-based schemes ([AC], [FAC], [EC], [FEC]) [12, 23, 24]. However, these are not employed in all cases due to diverse causes, among these is cardiovascular comorbidity [12, 25, 26].

Efficacy of Primary Chemotherapy

IBC appears to be a chemosensitive neoplasm. Retrospective analysis of some series permits the observation of a therapeutic response rate (RR) of 35–82 %, while pathological complete response (pCR) is identified in 6–37 %; these numbers have been observed with the use of anthracycline-based CT schemes [6, 13, 19, 23, 25] (Table 8.1). The use of taxanes in IBC has improved the pCR rate and progression-free survival (PFS) in comparison with schemes lacking these agents [26].

Three prospective, comparative studies have evaluated the efficacy of CT in IBC. The phase III Neoadjuvant Herceptin (NOAH) study included patients with noninflammatory locally advanced breast carcinoma (LABC) (T3, N1) and women with IBC (T4d), both groups HER2-positive, who received ten cycles of CT (doxorubicin and paclitaxel three cycles, followed by paclitaxel 175 mg for four cycles, and three cycles with CMF) followed by surgery (mastectomy) and RT. Patients were divided into two groups; the first received trastuzumab simultaneously, and the second did not receive this monoclonal antibody. The efficacy and safety results were compared with those of an HER2-negative control group. Event-free survival at 3 years was 71 % in those with HER2-positive and therapy with trastuzumab in comparison with 56 % in the HER2-negative group; this effect translated into a 41 % reduction in risk of recurrence, progression, or death. The benefits were observed in all of the subgroups, including those with IC. Overall survival (OS) at 3 years was 87 % with HER2-positive and trastuzumab and 79 % with HER2-negative. The pCR rate in breast, axilla, and both sites was higher in those treated with trastuzumab; the authors concluded that trastuzumab should be added to neoadjuvant CT in the presence of overexpression of HER2 [27].

The second clinical assay, (GeparTrio), compared the efficacy and safety of the combination of docetaxel, doxorubicin, and cyclophosphamide (TAC) during 6–8 cycles in 98 women with IBC, 194 with noninflammatory LABC, and 1,777 with operable cancer. Clinical response was 71 % for IBC, 69.6 % for the noninflammatory variant, and 83.4 % in operable cancer. pCR was similar between the two primary groups, 8.6 and 11.3 % ($p=0.542$), while this was observed in 17.7 % of those with operable cancer. Additionally, the pCR rate was higher in cases of women with IBC who received 8 cycles of CT in relation with those treated with six cycles, 17.2 versus 3.2 %, respectively ($p=0.103$). Histological grade was the unique predictor factor of pCR in cases with IBC and noninflammatory disease; when the three groups were combined, predictor factors comprised young age, non-lobular histology, histological grade 3, and negative hormonal receptors. The authors concluded that there is no difference in the RR to neoadjuvant CT [28].

The third clinical assay is the SWOG0012 study. It was designed to compare neoadjuvant CT with standard-scheme doxorubicin and cyclophosphamide during five cycles followed by weekly paclitaxel × 12 weeks versus metronomic therapy with weekly doxorubicin and oral cyclophosphamide daily during 15 weeks followed by paclitaxel weekly during 12 weeks. The assay included patients with noninflammatory and inflammatory locally advanced carcinoma. In the assay, neutropenia and febrile neutropenia was observed more frequently with the conventional scheme, while the metronomic therapy was more often associated with stomatitis, pharyngitis, and hand-foot syndrome; also, 35 % of the standard and 10 % of the experimental treatment arm developed grade 4 toxic effects. In the conventional treatment, the pCR rate observed was 20.7 %, while this was 24.3 % for metronomic therapy. pCR with IBC was 13 % with the standard scheme and 27 % in the metronomic one. PFS was not different in those with IBC treated with the standard or the experimental scheme, 28 versus 33 events, nor were there differences between the groups with IBC and noninflammatory disease with regard to OS and PFS [24].

Prevalence of Recurrent Disease

The recurrence of IBC is very frequent despite the high proportion of successfully treated cases and the improvement in survival expectancy generated by multimodal therapy. There is scarce information published on the frequency with which recurrent disease presents, as well as on the anatomic sites that it affects [6, 11, 12, 19, 22, 23, 25, 29]. Recurrence of IBC has been registered in 61–78 % [6, 11, 19, 22, 23]; when IBC recurrence presents, it has been identified as occurring at the locoregional level in 20–24 %, at a distance in 35–39 %, while affectation of both sites, locoregional and systemic, is informed as between 7 and 20 %; CNS involvement is reported between 7 and 9 % (Table 8.2).

Apparently, IBC recurrence is higher in comparison with noninflammatory breast cancer stage IIIA and/or IIB (72 vs. 54% and 77 %, respectively) [29]. Cristofanilli et al. [25] inform that among 240 cases recruited in five clinical trials of neoadjuvant CT followed by RT and/or mastectomy, recurrence was observed in 68 %, while this was detected in 51 % of cases with noninflammatory cancer; in this study, the frequency of systemic recurrence (visceral and bone) was similar in both groups (40.8 vs. 39.9 %), but local recurrence was greater in women affected by the inflammatory variant (15.4 vs. 7.0 %). On the other hand, the sequence of multimodal therapy appears to be a factor that exerts an influence on the recurrence pattern of this disease; a retrospective study informed that IBC recurrence is higher when mastectomy is employed as initial therapy in comparison with neoadjuvant CT; among 106 cases treated with neoadjuvant CT, 65.1 % were identified with recurrence, principally distant, while in 22 treated with mastectomy, recurrence was observed in 72.7 %, and locoregional and/or systemic dissemination was similar in this group (36 %) [12].

Recurrence Sites and Time of Presentation

Few reports include a detailed description of the anatomic sites affected by IBC recurrence. In reference to the spectrum of locoregional, distant, and CNS involvement, four reports have presented their observations [11, 14, 15, 23]. At the

Table 8.2 Prevalence and patterns of recurrence in inflammatory breast cancer

Author	*N*	Treatment	% patients with recurrence	% patients with LR	% patients with systemic recurrence	% patients with recurrence at both sites	% patients with recurrence in CNS en
Galmarini [11]	18	IBC IIIB neo CT→RT/Mx	78	7	93	NR	7
Liaw [22]	56	Trimodal	61	2	39	20	NR
Baldini [19]	68	neo CT→RT/Mx	73.5	20.6	35.3	7.4	NR
Labidi [6]	100	neo CT→RT/mx	71	24	37	10	NR
Ueno [23]	178	neo CT→RT/Mx	68	20	39	NR	9
Low [29]	46	BC	72	17	43	11	NR
	48	NI-BC IIIA	54	4	40	10	NR
	13	NI-BC IIIB	77	15	54	8	NR
Smooth [12]	106	neo CT→RT/Mx	65.1	19	36	NR	7
	22	Mx→CT/RT	72.7	36	36	NR	
Cristofanilli [26]	831	NI-BC	51.6	7.0	39.9	NR	NR
		neo CT→Mx/RT	68	15.4	40.8	NR	NR
	240	BC					
		neo CT→Mx/RT					

N number of patients, *NR* not reported, *LR* local recurrence, *CNS* central nervous system, *IBC* inflammatory breast cancer, *BC* breast carcinoma, *CT* chemotherapy, *RT* radiotherapy, neo *CT* neoadjuvant chemotherapy, *RT* radiotherapy, *Mx* mastectomy, *NI-BC* noninflammatory breast cancer

locoregional level, affectation of the chest wall is reported in 10 %, followed by affectation of the skin, while at the systemic level, the most frequently involved sites are liver, bone, lung, and soft tissues (Table 8.3). On the other hand, time to recurrent disease has been analyzed retrospectively in some series; in these reports, it is indicated that the average time is <2 years once multimodal therapy is concluded [6, 12, 18, 22].

Only two studies have been directed toward attempting to determine the frequency of disease presentation in its metastatic phase and the localization of the metastasis at the time of diagnosis. A study determined clinical stage through evaluation with computed axial tomography [14] and the other with positron emission tomography/(PET)/computed axial tomography [15]. Mvere et al. [14] detected stage IV in 26 %; the sites affected were lung and pleura, 11 %, respectively, and lymph node in 8 %. PET/computed axial tomography appears to be a more sensitive method for detecting the presence of metastatic activity in these cases. Carkaci et al. [15], in 41 cases, detected metabolic hyperuptake in the breast in 9 % and standard uptake value (SUV), 11.4 (range, 2.5–30.6), as well as in thickened skin, SUV 5.2 (range, 2.5–29.0). Twenty patients (49 %) had metastasis on diagnosis; the zones detected by PET/computed axial tomography were contralateral axillary lymph nodes 17 %, mediastinal 24 %, bone 22 %, and liver 15 %. In addition, in all cases considered in the locally advanced phase, in 44 %, affectation was noted in subpectoral lymph nodes, in 15 % in supraclavicular, and in 22 %, internal mammary lymph nodes.

On the other hand, IBC dissemination to CNS has been described in three retrospective reports [11, 12, 23]; its frequency was described as between 7 and 9 %. Recently, a study on the characteristics and prognosis of women with metastatic IBC to CNS was published [30]. A group of 203 women were evaluated at the MD Anderson Cancer Center (MDACC) in Houston, Texas; 40.4 % of these were found in stage IV, 29.6 % had a +/HER2-hormonal receptor phenotype, 34.5 % had HER2-positive, and 36 %, triple-negative. The mean time interval between diagnosis and detection of metastasis to CNS was 19 months, with an accumulated incidence at 1 and 2 years of 1.6 and 5.7 %, respectively; this was greater in those with

Table 8.3 Anatomical sites affected by metastasis at diagnosis and on recurrence of inflammatory carcinoma

Anatomical site/reference	At diagnosis % involved	At recurrence % involved
Liver [11, 15, 23]	12.5–15	10–22
Bone [11, 15, 23]	12.5–22	22
Lung [11, 14, 23]	11	6–14
Pleura [14, 23]	11	4
Central nervous system [11, 12, 23]		7–9
Soft tissues [11]		28
Mediastinal lymph nodes [14]	24	
Supraclavicular lymph nodes [11, 14, 23]	4.5–62.5	
Skin [11, 23]	12.5	4
Nonspecific lymph nodes [14]	8	
Axillary lymph nodes [15]	34	
Subpectoral lymph nodes [15]	44	
Internal mammary lymph nodes [15]	22	
Chest wall [23]		10
Contralateral breast [23]		2

stage IV at diagnosis. No associated factors were detected on development of metastatic activity. +/ HER2-negative hormonal receptor phenotype had a lesser risk than triple-negative [HR, 0.55; $p=0.24$], and the HER2-positive phenotype had a greater risk of metastasis than the triple-negative [HR, 1.02; $p=0.97$]; OS after identification of dissemination to CNS was 6 months.

Prognostic Factors of Recurrence

For LABC, the most important prognostic factor is the pCR to neoadjuvant CT. González et al. [31] evaluated the predictive factors of the distant development of metastasis in women with locally advanced carcinoma treated with neoadjuvant CT with anthracyclines and taxanes. Two groups were formed; in group 1, 266 women were included, 25 of these with IBC, and in group 2, there were 201 women, and those with the inflammatory variant were excluded. Average follow-up was 63 months. In all, there were 31 cases with distant metastasis; the 10-year metastasis-free rate was 82 %. Development of metastasis was associated with young age (<50 years), premenopausal status [HR, 3.08; $p=0.04$], inoperable disease (IIIB, IIIC, T4d) [HR, 4.24; $p < 0.0001$], and <10 axillary lymph nodes examined [HR, 2.94; $p=0.004$]. The authors created an algorithm in terms of the presence of one or several of these factors; the metastasis-free rate with 0 factors was 97, 88 % with one, 77 % with two, and 33 % with three factors.

Likewise, for IBC, the majority of reports coincide on that pCR (in breast and/or lymph nodes) represents the most important prognostic factor for recurrence. Panedes et al. [13], among 148 cases treated with primary CT followed by mastectomy, detected that 10-year locoregional RFS was associated with pCR. Harris et al. [21] observed local or regional failure in 47 % of cases in which pCR was achieved, while this was 74 % in those who did not achieve it; 5- and 10-year RFS was 45 and 27 % for treated women who did not achieve pCR, while assessments of these same parameters were 59 and 51 % in the presence of pCR. Other additional publications have assessed the prognostic effect of pCR [19, 25, 29].

The relevance of the pathological response in the lymph nodes was analyzed at the MDACC, where 61 cases with IBC and cytological diagnosis of axillary lymph-node metastasis received anthracycline- and/or taxane-based primary CT. pCR was registered in 14 patients (23 %) at the lymph-node level and in 13 patients (21 %) at the axillary and mammary level. Five-year OS without axillary response was 37 % in comparison with 82.5 % for those who did have pCR ($p=0.01$); the prognostic effect of pCR also exerted an influence on 5-year RFS, found to be 25 and 78.6 %, respectively. In the multivariate analysis, pCR showed a 0.18-times risk of death and a 0.09-times risk of recurrence ($p=0.03$ and $p=0.003$), respectively [32]. However, even in patients who achieved pCR, recurrence and death were observed in up to 33 % of cases [29].

Other factors that correlate with IBC recurrence are hormonal receptor state [12, 18, 25], presence of metastasis at diagnosis [18] or lymph-node disease at diagnosis [12, 25], and intensity of the CT scheme employed [33].

Locoregional Recurrent Disease

The incidence of locoregional recurrence is nearly 13 % [34] and is defined as the recurrence of a tumor in a mammary zone that was previously submitted to surgery or radiation [35]. After mastectomy, 10–20 % of cases experience locoregional recurrence, which produces pain, ulceration, bleeding, edema in the arm, or plexopathy in up to 62.5 % of cases. Many of these patients developed distant metastasis (81–93 %) within a lapse of 12–30 months [36], and 80 % of these patients died within a lapse of 2 years [37]. Ten-year OS and disease-free survival (DFS) in the presence of disease recurrence at the locoregional level has been estimated at 7–12 and at 22–26 %, respectively [34].

To date, no consensus exists on the management of locoregional recurrence; in a survey carried out in 494 oncologists, of whom 332 responded to the questionnaire (100 surgeons, 113 radiotherapists, and 107 medical oncologists), the responders considered locoregional recurrence as an affectation of the skin of the chest wall, the surgical scar, and the ipsilateral lymph nodes, as well as recurrence in the ipslateral breast. The majority of survey responders recommended surgery for resection of recurrence in the breast (99 %), scar (96 %), axillary lymph nodes (90 %), and chest wall (86 %), while resection was sparsely recommended in cases of involvement of the infraclavicular, supraclavicular, cervical, and internal mammary-chain lymph nodes. Also, 57 % of the physicians who responded to the survey recommended extended RT for treating the recurrence; 85 % suggested the utilization of systemic therapy if this has not already been applied, and 97 % were in agreement on modifying the systemic treatment scheme [34].

In the presence of isolated recurrence to chest wall, extensive surgical resection can be indicated; some reports indicate a 5-year survival rate of 43 % [37]. Chest-wall resection has been employed with the intention of palliating the symptoms and improving the patient's quality of life (QOL). Few studies have reported the results of this treatment type. A retrospective analysis of 15 women who underwent chest-wall, wide-margin resection, with total or partial sternectomy, reconstruction with rigid prosthesis of Marlex, and plastic reconstruction with muscular flap and vascularized peduncle, has been reported [38]. Radicality was reached in 73 % of cases; there were minor complications in 20 % and no major complications were observed; the stay in intensive care unit was 0.7 days, and there were 9.4 days of postsurgical hospital stay. At 25 months of follow-up, 40 % of the patients were alive (six patients) and disease-free; DFS at 1 and 2 years was 77 and 38 %, respectively, while OS was 71.4 and 29.7 %, respectively; the patients referred improvement in appearance and QOL.

The usefulness of full-thickness chest-wall resection to treat locoregional, post-RT recurrence and mastectomy was analyzed in a second report with 51 cases; the disease-free interval (DFI) was 70.3 months and follow-up, 29.4 months. Complete resection of the recurrence was obtained in all cases, but only one of the cases was catalogued as R1 and in six cases, the resection was classified as R2. Hospital mortality was 2 %, while complications were registered in 33 % (17 cases); these complications comprised bleeding in 14 %, flap necrosis in 3.9 %, wound infection in 7.8 %, and isolated cases of respiratory or myocardial failure, recurrent nerve paralysis, and empyema. Five-and 10-year OS was 41.4, 28.5, and 21.3 %, with a median of 50.1 months. Survival related factors by multivariate analysis were age at time of initial treatment [HR, 6.1; 95 % confidence interval [95 % CI, 1.9–19; $p=0.002$], bone infiltration [HR, 2.8; 95 % CI, 1.0–7.3; $p=0.04$], and DFI [HR, 2.6; 95 % CI, 0.9–7.6; $p=0.08$] [35].

The great majority of women with IBC who developed locoregional recurrence had previously received RT as part of initial multimodal therapy; unfortunately for these patients, the possibility of control by means of RT is lower due to the limitations of scaling the dose of radiation and the reduced tolerance of the tissues [36]. Thermoradiotherapy plus hyperthermia plus RT has been the standard treatment for unresectable recurrent lesions in previously irradiated zones. A retrospective study assessed the long-term results and the toxicity of re-irradiation and reoperation in 42 patients with locoregional recurrence; all of these were treated by a new surgical resection. Twelve received RT, while hyperthermia was applied in 21 cases with narrow resection margins and as part of the definitive treatment in unresectable cases. Five-year local control was 62 %, distant DFS was 57%, DFS was 44 %, and OS was 59 %. Better results were observed when re-irradiation was carried out at the first recurrence, 71 versus 40 %, when the case was operable, 75 versus 24 %, with R0 resection (80, 69, and 29 % respectively), and in the absence of lymph-node metastases, 73 versus 41 % [39].

An analysis of 39 cases with recurrent disease treated with thermoradiotherapy shows 1- and 2-year local control of 89 % and recurrence, 71 and 46 %, respectively; there were better results with micro- than with macroscopy recurrent disease [40]. Another report evaluated the role of thermoradiotherapy in two groups: group 1, 33 after narrow-surgical margin mastectomy, R1 resection, and high-risk breast cancer (T3/4, >3 affected lymph nodes grade 2/3); none received RT prior to thermoradiotherapy. In group 2, there were 37 women with chest-wall recurrence, which was R1-resected with residual or narrow-margin microscopy, <1 cm; 18 of these had received RT previously. At 36 months, OS, local control, and PFS in groups 1 and 2 were 90 and 89, 75 and 81, and 64 and 69 %, respectively; acute cutaneous toxicity was acceptable [41]. Finally, the use of RT, thermotherapy, and CT with epirubicin and ifosfamide has been explored in a study with 25 patients (14 with noninflammatory and 11 with inflammatory carcinoma); analysis showed an RR of 80 % and CR, 44 %. The authors observed a higher RR in patients who received RT with hyperfractionation in comparison with the conventional scheme (94 vs. 50 %), and in those with noninflammatory carcinoma (92 vs. 61 %), local and systemic toxicity was moderate [36].

Management of Brain Metastases

Brain metastases (BM) are present in 10–16 % of women with breast cancer, but in an autopsy series, their incidence reached up to 30 %. The interval between diagnosis of the primary tumor and identification of the metastases ranges between 2 and 3 years. Generally, BM present late, after identification of other metastatic sites such as lung and liver. Some factors that have been considered as predictive of the development of metastases to CNS (CNSM) are young age, overexpressed HER2, positive epidermal growth factor receptor (EGF), and positive lymph nodes; breast tumors with the triple-negative immunophenotype are associated more frequently with BM, while the incidence reaches 35 % in the presence of neoplasms that overexpress or amplify HER2. BM possess hematogenous dissemination. Seventy-eight percent of cases have multiple metastases, 14 % a solitary lesion, and 8 %, involvement of the leptomeninges [42–44].

By means of the results of the retrospective analysis of a series of cases, the behavior of metastatic brain lesions is demonstrated. Arslan et al. [45], among 259 cases with CNSM with primary localization in breast, detected locally advanced carcinoma in 25.7 %, with stage IV, 9 %, ductal histological variety in 91.7 %, histological grade III in 51.5 %, and premenopausal age in 66.2 %. CNSM were the first site of dissemination in 14.1 % of the cases; additionally, the lesion was documented in 22.4 % of cases, while multiple parenchymatous lesions were identified in 77.6 %; on the other hand, only 8 % of cases with leptomeningeal-level localized lesions. The breast carcinoma→metastasis interval was 31 months.

Diagnosis is based on the symptoms and the findings of neuroimaging studies, such as computed axial tomography and/or magnetic resonance imaging (MRI); at present, MRI is known as the most sensitive method for detection of metastatic lesions to CNS. The most frequent signs and symptoms are alterations in walking in 24 %, convulsions in 23 %, cephalea in 16 %, cognitive dysfunction in 14 %, nausea and vomiting in 11 %, cranial nerve dysfunction in 10 %, cerebellar symptoms in 2 %, and alterations in language in 2 %. Metastases in cerebellum can generate ataxia, cranial neuropathies, upper motor neuron dysfunction, hydrocephalus, cephalea, memory loss, and behavioral alterations [42, 43].

Medical treatment comprises the stabilization of edema-associated acute neurological symptoms, as well as convulsion control. For control of convulsive activity, dexamethasone and anticonvulsants are employed, such as phenytoin, carbamazepine, or valproic acid. In the treatment of BM, RT to holocranium is used, which is considered the treatment standard; the utilization of 30 Gy in ten fractions is commonly administered. Surgery is utilized to obtain symptom relief, local control, and confirmation of the diagnosis; generally, surgery is restricted to the treatment of isolated, accessible lesions. Stereotactic radiosurgery offers advantages such as low bleeding risk, low risk of infection, and low cost, because it does not require hospitalization. CT possesses limited value for BM [42, 43]. Recently, molecular biology has discovered the epidermal growth factor receptor pathway, the hexokinase HK2, integrin $\alpha v\beta 3$, HER2, and angiogenesis as elements involved in the genesis of metastases, and value has been conferred on these as potential therapeutic targets [44].

Unfortunately, expectations of survival are limited in women affected by the dissemination of breast carcinoma to CNS. Mean survival from diagnosis of metastases is 2–16 months and depends on the extracranial disease extension and the treatment applied. One-year survival is 20 months [42]. In the series of Arslan et al. [45], OS after diagnosis of brain metastases was 7.8 months and shorter for triple negatives, for which only 6.6 months was calculated. For cases in which surgical resection of the lesion is feasible, survival of 16 months has been reported, while for cases treated with RT, survival was 4.2 months [42, 43].

Treatment for Systemic Recurrence

The high frequency of systemic recurrence, at least in the 2 years after concluding multimodal therapy, in women with IBC who were exposed to anthracyclines and taxanes during the neoadjuvant CT phase obliges the consideration of development of pharmacological resistance. Resistance to chemotherapeutic agents can be generated from different mechanisms, including alterations in pharmacokinetics and metabolism, modifications in the target expression of the agent, compartmentalization of the drug in cellular organelles, drug-induced alterations in DNA damage repair, and expression of proteins that directly affect the cellular transport of drugs.

Some proteins involved in the development of resistance to antitumor agents are the following: *P-glycoprotein*, expressed in 40–66 % of breast cancers; multiple-drug-resistant protein type 1 (*MDR1*), which intervenes in resistance to vinca alkaloids, anthracyclines, and methotrexate; *breast cancer-resistant protein* (*BCRP*), involved in the cellular expulsion of diverse agents such as mitoxantrone, anthracyclines, methotrexate, and topoisomerase I inhibitors; and the *lung resistance-related protein* (*LRP*)/major vault protein related with cytoskeletal intracellular transport. Other mechanisms of resistance to antineoplastic agents implicate *microtubule alterations*, which are related with resistance to taxanes, such as the altered forms of β-tubulin as well as of the βIII subunit. In addition, changes in MAP4 and MAP-tau have been related with control of sensitivity to taxanes and vinca alkaloids. *DNA repair enzymes* have been related with resistance to anthracycline and epipodophyllotoxins, while some enzymes, such as aldehyde dehydrogenases ALDHA1 and ALDHA3, can catalyze the detoxification of cyclophosphamide [46, 47].

Resistance to anthracyclines and taxanes can be clinically defined as recurrent disease within the first 6 months after completing adjuvant or neoadjuvant CT that occurs during treatment, or the reappearance of the disease within the first 3 months of the last treatment dose [48]. It is considered that >90 % of treatment failures are due to pharmacological resistance. In the presence of advanced anthracycline- and/or taxane-resistant disease, there are limited therapeutic options. When this presents several years after therapy with anthracyclines and/or taxanes, use can be repeated with these agents, while if the recurrence takes place in <12 months, the use is preferred of other agents [49].

Antineoplastic Agents for Recurrent Breast Cancer Previously Treated with Anthracyclines and/or Taxanes

Currently, diverse antineoplastic agents to treat recurrent or metastatic breast cancer pretreated with anthracyclines and/or taxanes are available, and among these we find the following: *pegylated liposomal doxorubicin, docetaxel, capecitabine, gemcitabine, vinorelbine, ixabepilone, eribulin, cisplatin, epirubicin, mitoxantrone, etoposide, cyclophosphamide, trastuzumab, and lapatinib* [8]. Selection of the drug to use depends on three main factors: the state of HER2 expression or amplification; the patient's physical functioning state, and the disease's metastatic pattern. Under these two headings, distinct therapeutic approaches have been considered: [1] cases with or without overexpressed HER2, [2] low-risk disease, and [3] rapidly progressive disease.

On the other hand, depending on the functional physical state as well as on the metastatic pattern, the employment has been proposed of therapy as unique agent in sequential form, or the combination of two drugs. For women with recurring or metastatic breast cancer previously treated with anthracyclines and/or taxanes, with low functional state, and low-risk metastatic pattern (metastasis to bone, skin, and soft tissues), a timely treatment is considered to be one with unique agent, while for women with adequate physical functional state and visceral affectation (hepatic or pulmonary), the use has been recommended of combined CT schemes. The combinations are used for the rapidly progressive disease with the intention of maximizing disease response and control [48, 49].

Among the antineoplastic agents utilized in therapy for recurrent breast cancer and pretreated with anthracyclines and/or taxanes, we find some whose mechanisms of action and RR as unique agent are depicted in Table 8.4. At present, the National Cancer Comprehensive Network (NCCN) [8] suggests four combined CT schemes that can be employed for treating patients with recurrent or metastatic breast cancer, previously treated with anthracyclines and/or taxanes; among these are ixabepilone/capecitabine, gemcitabin/paclitaxel, gemcitabine/docetaxel, or docetaxel/capecitabine. The efficacy results that have been reported in randomized clinical assays for these four combinations, as well as for others that have been assayed during the past 10 years, are presented in Table 8.5 [50–63]. None of these assays have been specifically directed toward evaluating efficacy and safety in women affected by inflammatory and recurrent breast cancer; in fact, the description of the cases studied in each assay does not specify the number of women with recurrent inflammatory carcinoma who were included in these assays.

The most important efficacy results in these studies allows to consider that combined CT offers greater efficacy in relation to ORR, time to progression, and OS in the presence of therapy as unique agent, although the differences are not statistically significant in all cases. However, the combination of these antitumor agents is related with greater frequency of hematological and non-hematological toxicity. Despite that the incidence of toxic effects qualified as grade 3 and 4, the authors in these studies consider the toxicity as manageable and reversible.

Currently, a sole study has been conducted to evaluate the therapeutic effects and the safety of lapatinib, a reversible inhibitor of EGFR and HER2, in IBC that is HER2-positive, recurrent, or progressive to therapy with the monoclonal antibody, trastuzumab. In this phase II study, the primary objective was to analyze the RR and secondly, to analyze the clinical benefit, PFS,

Table 8.4 Antitumor agents utilized in the treatment of anthracycline- and/or taxane-resistant breast cancer

Agent	Class	Mechanism of action	RR, mono-drug (%)
Capecitabine	Antimetabolite	Inhibits DNA synthesis and interferes in RNA transcription	20–36
Gemcitabine	Antimetabolite	Inhibits DNA synthesis and autopotentiation	14–37
Docetaxel	Inhibitor of microtubules	Inhibits microtubular depolymerization	18–68
Paclitaxel	Inhibitor of microtubules	Inhibits microtubular depolymerization	17–54
Vinorelbine	Vinca alkaloid	Inhibits microtubule formation	25–47
Ixabepilone	Epothilone analog	Stabilizes the microtubule dynamic	11.5–57
Eribulin	Inhibitor of microtubules	Suppresses microtubular polymerization	9.3–21
Albumin-bound paclitaxel	Inhibitor of microtubules	Inhibits microtubular depolymerization	14–48
Trastuzumab	Recombinant monoclonal antibody	Inhibition of HER2	12–34
Lapatinib	Inhibitor of TK, small-molecule	Inhibition of HER2 and EGFR	9–47

RR response rate, *DNA* deoxyribonucleic acid, *TK* tyrosine-kinase, *HER2* human epidermal growth factor receptor-2, *EGFR* epidermal growth factor receptor

Table 8.5 Efficacy results in comparative clinical assays of chemotherapy in breast cancer previously treated with anthracyclines and/or taxanes

Author	Treatment arm	*N*	ORR (%)	Progression (%)	TTP (months)	OS months
O'Shaugnessy [50]	Docetaxel/capecitabine	255	42	11	6.1	14.5
	Docetaxel	256	30	20	4.2	11.5
Albain [51]	Gemcitabine/paclitaxel	266	43.1	NR	6.1	18.6
	Paclitaxel	263	26.9	NR	3.9	15.8
Thomas [52]	Ixabepilone/capecitabine	375	33	15	5.8	NR
	Capecitabine	377	14	27	4.8	NR
Miller [53]	Bevacizumab/capecitabine	232	19.8	NR	4.8	15.1
	Capecitabine	230	9.1	NR	4.1	14.5
Gray [54]	Bevacizumab/paclitaxel	368	48.9	91.3	11.3	NR
	Paclitraxel	354	22.2	90.2	5.8	NR
Robert [55]	Placebo/capecitabine	206	23.6	NR	5.7	NR
	Bevacizumab/capecitabine	409	35.4	NR	8.6	NR
	Placebo/anthracy-cline/taxane	207	37.9	NR	8.0	NR
	Bevacizumab/anthracycline/taxane	415	51.3	NR	9.2	NR
Martin [56]	Gemcitabine/vinorelbine	123	36	32	6.0	15
	Vinorelbine	125	26	46	4.0	16.4

(continued)

Table 8.5 (continued)

Author	Treatment arm	*N*	ORR (%)	Progression (%)	TTP (months)	OS months
Chan [57]	Gemcitabine/ docetaxel	153	32	13	4.2	19.2
	Docetaxel/ capecitabine	152	32	14	4.0	21.4
Stemmler [58]	Gemcitabine/ vinorelbine	46	39	26.8	5.7	17.5
	Gemcitabine/ cisplatin	45	47.7	25.0	6.9	13.0
	Gemcitabine/ capecitabine	50	34.7	24.5	8.3	19.4
Cortes [59]	Eribulin	508	12	41	3.7	13.1
	Other	254	5	49	2.2	10.6
Barrios [60]	Sunitinib	238	11	NR	6.9	15.3
	Capecitabine	244	16	NR	9.3	24.6
Sparano [61]	Ixabepilone/ capecitabine	609	43.3	12	6.2	14.0
	Capecitabine	612	28.8	24	4.4	11.3
Geyer [62]	Lapatinib/ capecitabine	163	22	NR	8.4	NR
	Capecitabine	161	14	NR	4.1	NR
Gradishar [63]	Albumin-bound paclitaxel	229	33	NR	5.2	16.2
	Conventional paclitaxel	225	19	NR	4.0	13.9

N number of patients, *ORR* objective response rate, *TTP* time to progression, *OS* overall survival, *NR* not reported

response time, and response duration, OS, and QOL. One hundred twenty-six women were treated with lapatinib at a dose of 1,500 mg/day orally; RR was 39 % by clinical evaluation, while this was observed in 15 % when Response Evaluation Criteria in Solid Tumors (RECIST) criteria were applied. Median PFS was 14.6 weeks, and PFS at 6 months was 22 %. During the assay, 112 cases progressed (88.9 %), and 80 deaths (63 %) were registered; median OS was 11.2 months. The authors noted greater OS in women considered as responders in comparison with those who did not show response to the tyrosine-kinase inhibitor, 18.4 versus 8.4 months, respectively. Duration of response was 20.9 weeks. The most frequent toxic effect was diarrhea, which was detected in 59 % of cases; other side effects included fatigue, nausea, cutaneous erythema, anorexia, dyspnea, vomiting, and grade 1–3 back pain. Serious adverse events presented in 32 %, with dyspnea, pleural hemorrhage, and fever the most frequent [64].

The Molecular Biology of Inflammatory Breast Cancer

The need for the availability of novel pharmacological agents for treating recurrent disease is urgent; thus, new approximations have been performed of clinical and translational research in terms of the biological behavior of IBC.

Nearly one-half of cases are classified as basal carcinomas and as HER2-positive, which partially explains the fatal evolution of inflammatory carcinoma. A study compared the immunohistochemical profile of 91 IBC and of 547 noninflammatory breast carcinomas. Estrogen receptors were negative in 53.8 versus 26.2 % ($p < 0.001$); progesterone receptor-negative, 52.8 versus 35.3 % ($p < 0.001$); HER2-positive, 33.3 versus 14.4 % ($p < 0.001$); CK14-positive, 19.1 versus 5.4 % ($p < 0.001$); P-cadherin-positive, 75.9 versus 48.1 % ($p < 0.001$); and positive expression of Ki-67 >20, 41.1 versus 12.9 % ($p < 0.001$). According to the criteria employed in the study to define molecular subtypes, cases with ER+/PR+ were designated as luminal carcinoma, HER2+ (HER2), and ER-negative/HER2-negative as double-negative or basal. The authors reported a prevalence of the molecular subtypes for all cases with inflammatory and noninflammatory carcinoma as follows: luminal, 33.8 versus 15.9 % ($p < 0.001$); basal, 33.3 versus 14.4 % ($p < 0.001$); and HER2, 29.3 versus 58.9 % ($p < 0.001$) [65].

Diverse pathological and immunohistochemical characteristics distinguish IBC, among these the presence of a high histological grade; high cellular proliferation rate; S-phase; aneuploidy; high expression level of p53, MUC1, RhoC, and E-cadherin; and positive expression of the epidermal growth factor receptor (HER2 and EGFR). In addition, the increased density of intratumor microvessels, angiogenesis, factors related with lymphangiogenesis, and endothelial vascular growth factor (VEGF-A, VEGF-C, VEGF-D, Flt-1, KDR, Tie-1, Tie-2) have been reported in this breast cancer variant [2, 66].

Also, some genes have been related with the aggressivity of inflammatory carcinoma, as follows: genes related with nuclear factor-kappa beta (NF-κB) associated with cellular migration, invasion, and metastasis and overexpression of Rho CGTPase, a member of the RAS family of GTP protein binders that regulate the angiogenic factors (VEGF, FCF), which promote cellular motility and invasion [2, 4].

The density grade of intratumor microvessels has been demonstrated to be greater in inflammatory carcinoma in comparison with noninflammatory locally advanced carcinoma, 25.5 versus 6.5. VEGF-inhibitor drugs have been created, such as bevacizumab, semaxanib, and pazopanib [17]. Some efforts have begun to evaluate the efficacy of certain antiangiogenic agents in inflammatory breast cancer. A study with 21 patients (20 with inflammatory and one with noninflammatory) evaluated the effects of bevacizumab associated with doxorubicin and docetaxel, in which an ORR was registered of 67 %, five with stable disease and two with progression; PFS was 25.3 months [67]. On the other hand, pazopanib is a small-molecule tyrosine-kinase inhibitor of VEGF-1, VEGF-2, VEGF-3, PDGFR alpha, PDGFR beta, and KIT. In 21 patients treated with 800 mg, orally, in 28-day cycles, an RR was observed of 1 % and of 55 % with stable disease [68].

Novel concepts and potential therapeutic targets for inflammatory carcinoma are arising; among these are the CXCR4 and CCR7 chemokine receptors, which function as neoangiogenesis mediators and of T cell differentiation. At the MDACC, the expression was investigated of both chemokines among 44 cases with inflammatory carcinoma; CXCR4-positive was detected in 40.9 % and CCR7-positive in 22.7 %, with positive expression in both of 18.2 %. Five-year OS in cases with CXCR4-positive was 24.8 % in comparison with 42.3 % observed for negative cases; in the presence of CCR7+, survival was less, at 20 versus 41.9 %, respectively [66].

Molecular targets in the vasculolymphatic process show greater potential in IBC, such as bevacizumab and semaxanib. Lapatinib blocks the EGFR and HER2, additional targets comprise WTN1 cell proliferation signaling pathway protein 3 (ISP2, Rho GTPase C-, and p27) and overexpression of E-cadherin, which is a mesenchymal epithelial transition (MET) marker. EGFR is expressed in 30 % of the inflammatory variety and is associated with high risk of recurrence [4, 69].

References

1. Globocan. International agency for research on cancer. 2008. Available at: http://www.dep.iarc.fr. Accesed July 2011.
2. Dushkin H, Cristofanilli M. Inflammatory breast cancer. J Natl Compr Canc Netw. 2011;9:233–41.
3. Anderson WF, Schairer C, Chen BE, Hance KW, Levine PH. Epidemiology of inflammatory breast cancer. Breast Dis. 2005;22:9–23.
4. Robertson FM, Bondy M, Yang W, Yamauchi H, Wiggins S, Kamrudin S, et al. Inflammatory breast cancer: the disease, the biology and the treatment. CA Cancer J Clin. 2010;60:351–75.
5. Chia S, Swain SM, Byrd DR, Mankoff DA. Locally advanced and inflammatory breast cancer. J Clin Oncol. 2008;26:786–90.
6. Labidi SI, Mrad K, Mezlini A, Ouarda MA, Combes JD, Ben Abdallah M, et al. Inflammatory

breast cancer in Tunisia in the era of multimodality therapy. Ann Oncol. 2008;19:473–80.
7. Hance KW, Anderson WF, Devesa SS, Young HA, Levine PL. Trends in inflammatory breast carcinoma incidence and survival: the surveillance and epidemiology and end results program at the National Cancer Institute. J Natl Cancer Inst. 2005;97:966–75.
8. National Comprehensive Cancer Network. Breast cancer. NCCN clinical practice guidelines in oncology. 2011; v.2. Available at: www.nccn.org. Accessed July 2011.
9. Edge SB, Byrd DR, Compton CC, Fritz AG, Greene FL, Trotti A, editors. AJCC cancer staging manual. 7th ed. Chicago: Springer; 2010.
10. Brooks HL, Mandava N, Pizzi WF, Shah S. Inflammatory breast carcinoma: a community hospital experience. J Am Coll Surg. 1998;186:622–9.
11. Galmarini CM, Garbovesky C, Galmarini D, Galmarini FC. Clinical outcome and prognosis of patients with inflammatory breast cancer. Am J Clin Oncol. 2002;25:172–7.
12. Smooth RL, Koch CA, Degnim AC, Sterioff S, Donohue JH, Grant CS, et al. A single-center experience with inflammatory breast cancer, 1985–2003. Arch Surg. 2006;141:567–73.
13. Panades M, Olivotto IA, Speers CH, Shenkier T, Olivotto TA, Weir L, et al. Evolving treatment strategies for inflammatory breast cancer: a population-based survival analysis. J Clin Oncol. 2005;23: 1941–50.
14. Mvere MZ, James JJ, Cornford EJ, Tannant SL, Evans AJ, Ellis IO, et al. Frequency and patterns of metastatic disease in locally advanced inflammatory and non-inflammatory breast cancer. Clin Oncol (R Coll Radiol). 2011;23:608–12.
15. Carkaci S, Macapinlac HA, Cristofanilli M, Mawlawi O, Rohren E, González AM, et al. Retrospective study of 18F-FDG PET/CT in the diagnosis of inflammatory breast cancer: preliminary data. J Nucl Med. 2009;50:231–8.
16. Dawood S, Merajver SD, Viens P, Vermeulen PB, Swain SM, Buchholz TA, et al. International expert panel on inflammatory breast cancer: consensus statement for standardized diagnosis and treatment. Ann Oncol. 2011;22:515–23.
17. Sinclair S, Swain SM. Primary systemic chemotherapy for inflammatory breast cancer. Cancer. 2010;116 Suppl 11:2821–8.
18. Sutherland S, Ashley S, Walsh G, Smith IE, Johnston SRD. Inflammatory breast cancer – The Royal Marsden Hospital experience. Cancer. 2010;116 Suppl 11:2815–20.
19. Baldini E, Gardin G, Evangelista G, Prochilo T, Collecchi P, Lionetto R. Long-term results of combined-modality therapy for inflammatory breast carcinoma. Clin Breast Cancer. 2004;5:358–63.
20. Goldfarb JM, Pippen JE. Inflammatory breast cancer: the experience of Baylor University Medical Center at Dallas. Proc (Bayl Univ Med Cent). 2011;24:86–8.
21. Harris E, Schultz D, Bertsch H, Fox K, Glick J, Solin LJ. Ten-year outcome after combined modality therapy for inflammatory breast cancer. Int J Radiat Oncol Biol Phys. 2003;55:1200–8.
22. Liaw SL, Benda RK, Morris CG, Mendenhall NP. Inflammatory breast carcinoma: outcomes with trimodality therapy for nonmetastatic disease. Cancer. 2004;100:920–8.
23. Ueno NT, Buzdar AU, Singletary SE, Ames FC, McNeese MD, Holmes FA, et al. Combined-modality treatment of inflammatory breast carcinoma: twenty years of experience at M.D. Anderson Cancer Center. Cancer Chemother Pharmacol. 1997;40:321–9.
24. Ellis GK, Barlow WE, Gralow JR, Hortobagyi GN, Rusell CA, Royce ME, et al. Phase III comparison of standard doxorubicin and cyclophosphamide versus weekly doxorubicin and daily oral cyclophosphamide plus granulocyte colony-stimulating factor as neoadjuvant therapy for inflammatory and locally advanced breast cancer: SWOG 0012. J Clin Oncol. 2011;29: 1014–21.
25. Cristofanilli M, Valero V, Buzdar AU, Broglio KR, González-Angulo AM, Sneige N, et al. Inflammatory breast cancer and patterns of recurrence. Cancer. 2007;110:1436–44.
26. Cristofanilli M, González-Angulo AM, Buzdar AU, Kau SW, Frye DK, Hortobagyi GN. Paclitaxel improves the prognosis in estrogen receptor-negative in inflammatory breast cancer: the M.D. Anderson Cancer Center experience. Clin Breast Cancer. 2004; 4:415–9.
27. Gianni L, Eiermann W, Semiglazov V, Manikhas A, Lluch A, Tjulandin S, et al. Neoadjuvant chemotherapy with trastuzumab followed by adjuvant trastuzumab versus neoadjuvant chemotherapy alone, in patients with HER2-positive locally advanced breast cancer (the NOAH trial): a randomized controlled superiority trial with a parallel HER2-negative cohort. Lancet. 2010;375:377–84.
28. Costa SD, Loibl S, Kaufmann M, Zahm DM, Huober J, Eidthmann H, et al. Neoadjuvant chemotherapy shows similar response in patients with inflammatory or locally advanced breast cancer when compared with operable breast cancer: a secondary analysis of the GeparTrio trial data. J Clin Oncol. 2010;28:83–91.
29. Low JA, Berman AW, Steinberg SM, Danforth DM, Lippman ME, Swain SM. Long-term follow-up for locally advanced and inflammatory breast cancer patients treated with multimodality therapy. J Clin Oncol. 2004;22:4067–74.
30. Dawood S, Ueno NT, Valero V, Andreopoulou E, Hsu L, Lara J, et al. Incidence and survival following brain metastases among women with inflammatory breast cancer. Ann Oncol. 2010;21:2348–55.
31. González-Angulo AM, McGuire SE, Buchholz TA, Tucker SL, Kuerer HM, Rouzier R, et al. Factors predictive of distant metastases in patients with breast cancer who have a pathologic complete response after

neoadjuvant chemotherapy. J Clin Oncol. 2005; 23:7098–104.
32. Hennessy BT, González-Angulo AM, Hortobagyi GN, Cristofanilli M, Kau SW, Broglio K, et al. Disease-free and overall survival after pathologic complete disease remission of cytologically proven inflammatory breast carcinoma axillary lymph node metastases after primary systemic chemotherapy. Cancer. 2006;106:1000–6.
33. Bertucci F, Tarpin C, Charaf-Jauffred E, Bardou VJ, Braud AC, Tallet A, et al. Multivariate analysis of survival in inflammatory breast cancer: impact of intensity of chemotherapy in multimodality treatment. Bone Marrow Transplant. 2004;33:913–20.
34. Clemons M, Hamilton T, Mansi J, Lockwood G, Goss P. Management of recurrent locoregional breast cancer: oncologist survey. Breast. 2003;12:328–37.
35. Friedel G, Kuipers T, Engel C, Schopf C, Veit S, Zoller J, et al. Full-thickness chest wall resection for locally recurrent breast cancer. Thorac Surg Sci 2005;2:Doc01.
36. Feyerabend T, Wiedemann GJ, Jäger B, Vesely H, Mahlmann B, Richter E. Local hyperthermia, radiation and chemotherapy in recurrent breast cancer is feasible and effective except for inflammatory disease. Int J Radiat Oncol Biol Phys. 2001;49:1317–25.
37. Wilson RE. Surgical management of locally advanced and recurrent breast cancer. Cancer. 1984;53:752–7.
38. Veronesi G, Scanagatta P, Goldhirsch A, Rietjens M, Colleoni M, Pelosi G, et al. Results of chest wall resection for recurrent or locally advanced breast malignancies. Breast. 2007;16:297–302.
39. Müller AC, Eckert F, Heinrich V, Bamberg M, Brucker S, Hehr T. Re-surgery and chest wall re-irradiation for recurrent breast cancer- a second curative approach. BMC Cancer. 2011;11:197–204.
40. Hehr T, Lamprecht U, Glocker S, Clasen J, Paulsen F, Budach W, et al. Thermoradiotherapy for locally recurrent breast cancer with skin involvement. Int J Hyperthermia. 2001;17:291–301.
41. Welz S, Hehr T, Lamprecht U, Scheithauer H, Budach W, Bamberg M. Thermoradiotherapy of the chest wall in locally advanced or recurrent breast cancer with marginal resection. Int J Hyperthermia. 2005;21:159–67.
42. Weil RJ, Palmieri DC, Bronder JL, Stark AM, Steeg PS. Breast cancer metastasis to the central nervous system. Am J Pathol. 2005;167:913–20.
43. Chang EL, Lo S. Diagnosis and management of central nervous system metastases from breast cancer. Oncologist. 2003;8:398–410.
44. Gril B, Evans L, Palmieri D, Steeg PS. Translational research in brain metastasis is identifying molecular pathways that may lead to the development of new therapeutic strategies. Eur J Cancer. 2010;46: 1204–10.
45. Arslan UY, Oksuzoglu B, Aksoy S, Harputlouglu H, Turker I, Ozisik Y, et al. Breast cancer subtypes and outcomes of central nervous system metastases. Breast. 2011;20:562–7.
46. Rivera E. Implications of anthracycline-resistant and taxane-resistant metastatic breast cancer and new therapeutic options. Breast J. 2010;16:252–63.
47. González-Angulo AM, Morales-Vázquez F, Hortobagyi GN. Overview of the resistance to the systemic therapy in patients with breast cancer. Adv Exp Med Biol. 2007;608:1–22.
48. Moreno-Aspitia A, Pérez EA. Treatment options for breast cancer resistant to anthracycline and taxane. Mayo Clin Proc. 2009;84:533–45.
49. Rivera E. Management of metastatic breast cancer. Monotherapy options for patients resistant to anthracyclines and taxanes. Am J Clin Oncol. 2010;33:176–85.
50. O'Shaughnessy J, Miles D, Vukelja S, et al. Superior survival with capecitabine plus docetaxel combination therapy in anthracycline-pretreated patients with advanced breast cancer: phase III trial results. J Clin Oncol. 2002;20:2812–23.
51. Albain KS, Nag SM, Calderillo-Ruíz G, et al. Gemcitabine plus paclitaxel versus paclitaxel monotherapy in patients with metastatic breast cancer and prior anthracycline treatment. J Clin Oncol. 2008;26: 3950–7.
52. Thomas ES, Gómez HL, Li RK, et al. Ixabepilone plus capecitabine for metastatic breast cancer progressing after anthracycline and taxane treatment. J Clin Oncol. 2007;25:5210–7.
53. Miller KD, Chap LI, Holmes FA, et al. Randomized phase III trial of capecitabine compared with bevacizumab plus capecitabine in patients with previously treated metastatic breast cancer. J Clin Oncol. 2005;23:792–9.
54. Gray R, Bhattacharya S, Bowden C, Miller K, Comis RL. Independent review of E2100: a phase III trial of bevacizumab plus paclitaxel versus paclitaxel in women with metastatic breast cancer. J Clin Oncol. 2009;27:4966–72.
55. Robert NJ, Diéras V, Glaspy J, Brufsky AM, Bondarenko I, Lipatov ON, et al. RIBBON-1: randomized, double-blind, placebo-controlled, phase III trial of chemotherapy with or without bevacizumab for first-line treatment of human epidermal growth factor receptor 2 negative, locally recurrent or metastatic breast cancer. J Clin Oncol. 2011;29: 1252–60.
56. Martin M, Ruiz A, Muñoz M, Balil A, García-Mata J, Calvo L, et al. Gemcitabine plus vinorelbine versus vinorelbine monotherapy in patients with metastatic breast cancer previously treated with anthracyclines and taxanes: final results of the phase III Spanish Breast Cancer Research Group (GEICAM) trial. Lancet Oncol. 2007;8:219–25.
57. Chan S, Romieu G, Huober J, Dolozier T, Tubiana-Hulin M, et al. Phase III study of gemcitabine plus docetaxel compared with capecitabine plus docetaxel for anthracycline-pretreated patients with metastatic breast cancer. J Clin Oncol. 2009;27:1753–60.
58. Stemmler HJ, diGiogia D, Freier W, Tessen HW, Gitsch G, Jonat W, et al. Randomised phase II trial of

gemcitabine plus vinorelbine vs gemcitabine plus cisplatin vs gemcitabine plus capecitabine in patients with pretreated metastatic breast cancer. Br J Cancer. 2011;104:1071–8.
59. Cortes J, O'Shaughnessy J, Loesch D, Blum JL, Vahdat LT, Petrakova K, et al. Eribulin monotherapy versus treatment of physician's choice in patients with metastatic breast cancer (EMBRACE): a phase III open-label randomized study. Lancet. 2011;377:914–23.
60. Barrios CH, Liu MC, Lee SC, Vanlemmens L, Ferrero JM, Tabei T, et al. Phase III randomized trial of sunitinib versus capecitabine in patients with previously treated HER2-negative advanced breast cancer. Breast Cancer Res Treat. 2010;121:121–31.
61. Sparano JA, Vrdoljak E, Rixe O, Xu B, Manikhas A, Medina C, et al. Randomized phase III trial of Ixabepilone plus capecitabine versus capecitabine in patients with metastatic breast cancer previously treated with an anthracycline and a taxane. J Clin Oncol. 2010;28:3256–63.
62. Geyer CE, Forster J, Lindquist T, Chan S, Romieu CG, Pienkowski T, et al. Lapatinib plus capecitabine for HER2-positive advanced breast cancer. N Engl J Med. 2006;355:2733–43.
63. Gradishar WJ, Tjulandin S, Davidson N, Shaw H, Desai N, Bhar P, et al. Phase III trial of nanoparticle albumin-bound paclitaxel compared with polyethylated castor oil-based paclitaxel in women with breast cancer. J Clin Oncol. 2005;23:7794–803.
64. Kaufman B, Trudeau M, Awada A, Blackwell K, Bachelot T, Salazar V, et al. Lapatinib monotherapy in patients with HER2-overexpressing relapsed or refractory inflammatory breast cancer: final results and survival of the expanded HER2+ in cohort EGF103009, a phase II study. Lancet Oncol. 2009;10:581–8.
65. Ben Hamida A, Labidi IS, Mrad K, Charaffe-Jauffret E, Ben Arab S, Esterni B, et al. Markers of subtypes in inflammatory breast cancer studied by immunohistochemistry: prominent expression of P-cadherin. BMC Cancer. 2008;8:28–35.
66. Cabioglu N, Gong Y, Islam R, Broglio KR, Sneige N, Sahin A, et al. Expression of growth factor and chemokine receptors: new insights in the biology of inflammatory breast cancer. Ann Oncol. 2007;18:1021–9.
67. Wedam SB, Low JA, Yang SX, Chow CK, Choyke P, Danforth D, et al. Antiangiogenic and antitumor effects of bevacizumab in patients with inflammatory and locally advanced breast cancer. J Clin Oncol. 2006;24:769–77.
68. Taylor SK, Chia S, Dent S, Clemons M, Agulnik M, Grenci P, et al. A phase II study of pazopanib in patients with recurrent or metastatic invasive breast carcinoma: a trial of the Princess Margaret Hospital Phase II Consortium. Oncologist. 2010;15:810–8.
69. Yamauchi H, Ueno NT. Targeted therapy in inflammatory breast cancer. Cancer. 2010;116 Suppl 11:2758–9.

The Molecular Biology of Inflammatory Breast Cancer

9

Horacio Astudillo-de la Vega, Erika Ruiz-Garcia, Paula Juarez-Sanchez, Jaime G. de la Garza-Salazar, and Oscar Gerardo Arrieta-Rodriguez

Introduction

Inflammatory breast cancer (IBC) is a rare and clinically more aggressive type of breast cancer. It is characterized by blockade of lymphatic vessels by cancerous cells in the skin of the breast. This type of breast cancer is called "inflammatory" because the breast often appears to be swollen, reddened, or "inflamed" [1]. It is diagnosed mainly in young women in comparison with other breast cancer types. African-American women have IBC at a younger age than Caucasian women. Some studies have demonstrated an association between familial history of breast cancer and IBC; however, additional studies are required to demonstrate this [2]. IBC is classified as breast cancer at stage IIIB or IV. IBC tends to grow rapidly and the physical appearance of the breast of patients with inflammatory cancer is different from that of patients with other stage III cancers [2].

H. Astudillo-de la Vega, M.D., M.Sc., Ph.D. (✉)
Laboratory of Translational Research in Cancer, Oncology Hospital, National Medical Center "Siglo XXI", Instituto Mexicano del Seguro Social (IMSS), Av. Cuauhtémoc 330, Col. Doctores, 06720 Mexico City, DF, Mexico
e-mail: hastud2@aol.com

E. Ruiz-Garcia
Department of Medical Oncology, Instituto Nacional de Cancerología-México (INCan), Secretaría de Salud (Ssa), Mexico City, DF, Mexico

P. Juarez-Sanchez, M.D.
Department of Pathology, Instituto Nacional de Cancerologia-Mexico (INCan), Ssa, Mexico City, DF, Mexico

J.G. de la Garza-Salazar, M.D.
Department of Clinical Investigation, Instituto Nacional de Cancerologia-Mexico, Mexico City, DF, Mexico

O.G. Arrieta-Rodriguez, M.D.
Department of Medical Oncology, Instituto Nacional de Cancerología-México (INCan), Secretaría de Salud (Ssa), Mexico City, DF, Mexico

The Role of Pro-inflammatory Cytokines and Chemokines in Inflammatory Breast Cancer

Cytokines are low-molecular-weight (LMW) regulatory proteins or glycoproteins that modulate the intensity and duration of the immune response, whether by stimulation or inhibition of the activation, proliferation, and/or differentiation of the target cell. Different cytokines are known to play diverse roles in the initiation and progression of breast cancer. Interleukin 10 (IL-10) is a pleiotropic anti-inflammatory cytokine that induces immunosuppression and that aids in escape from immune surveillance. Similarly to other cytokines, IL-10 can be exercising a proliferative as well as inhibitory dual effect on breast tumor cells, demonstrating the complex role of IL-10 in breast cancer initiation and progression [3]. Recently, the IL-6 inflammatory cytokine has been reported as a potential inducer of the mesenchymal-epithelial

J.G. de la Garza-Salazar et al. (eds.), *Inflammatory Breast Cancer*,
DOI 10.1007/978-0-85729-991-8_9, © Springer-Verlag London 2013

transition (MET) in epithelial-phenotype breast cancer; even more so, MET induced "stem cell" characteristics in normal and transformed breast cells [4]. There is evidence that IL-6 is capable of generating CD44+ cells with "stem cell"-like properties through MET induction. The existing relationship has been demonstrated between an IL-6 inflammatory cytokine and "stem cell"-like breast cancer cells, although MET appears to comprise a critical mechanism for the production of "stem cell"-like cancerous cells [4]. By means of genetic expression studies, it was reported that estrogen receptor (ER)-negative IBC subtypes are characterized by overexpression of nuclear kappa beta factor (*NFkB*) target genes [5]. It was previously known that *NFkB* and the target genes associated with their stimulation are involved in tumor progression. Thus, the potential use has been explored of curcumin and its analogs, as well as of the inhibitor of bortezomib proteasome degradation (Velcade®), because these are capable of inhibiting *NFkB*. Some studies have also demonstrated correlation among *NFkB* activation, toll-like receptors (TLR), and hyperactivation of the mitogenic activator protein-kinase (MAPK) signaling pathway, which could be linked with the overexpression of the epithelial growth factor receptor (EGFR) and/or human epithelial growth factor receptor-2 (HER2). Other studies have demonstrated the co-expression of EGFR and the CXCR4 chemokine receptors of IBC and have demonstrated a significant association with diminution in global survival (GS) [6]. These signaling pathways undoubtedly provide novel therapeutic targets for developing IBC inhibitors.

Molecular Factors of Obesity, Inflammation, and Lactation Associated with Inflammatory Breast Cancer

Weight increase and obesity have been identified as a risk and important prognostic factor for breast cancer in postmenopausal women. Several hypotheses have been proposed to explain the association of obesity with postmenopausal breast cancer. Specific obesity-associated factors, such as leptin, insulin, and inflammatory mediators, have been observed to exert an influence on the prognosis of mammary cancer growth independently of and at least in part due to the interaction of the estrogenic signaling pathway at a cellular level. Therefore, the use of anti-inflammatory and antidiabetic drugs associated with conventional hormonal therapies and interventions in physical activity and diet could provide a new therapeutic application for inflammatory and noninflammatory breast cancer [7]. Another novel concept utilized to describe the increase in the pro-inflammatory systemic state is inflamm-aging. This novel concept of inflammation and aging is the product of a disruption in the cytokine networks that regulate the inflammatory response, in which stromal "stem cells" and stromal fibroblasts become pro-inflammatory cytokine-producer cells produced by the accumulation of DNA damage. Inflamm-aging propagates the capacity of pro-inflammatory cytokines to ignite response to DNA damage in the healthy cells that surround DNA-damaged cells. Macrophages are the main actors in the inflamm-aging phenomenon, amplifying the phenomenon by means of the action of transmitting pro-inflammatory signals to local as well as to systemic levels. Thus, it is clear that the inflammatory stage induced directly or indirectly, together with age or the aging process, should contribute to increasing the incidence of cancer, particularly in states of inflammatory origin [8]. Visceral adiposity and the metabolic syndrome (Me Sy) have now been related with carcinogenesis. The relation between obesity and cancer has been demonstrated in a large amount of epidemiologically well-designed studies. Visceral adipose tissue is already recognized as an important secretor of factors that systemically alter the endocrine, metabolic, and immunological state toward carcinogenesis; thus, an excess of this tissue gives rise to a state of chronic systemic inflammation with associated insulin resistance and metabolic alterations, a state commonly known as Me Sy. An increase has been demonstrated in the risks of having cancer of the breast, colon, and esophagus due to maintaining this Me Sy state and visceral adiposity. In addition, these two factors have been associated with tumor progression and a reduction in survival. The molecular mechanisms of how these two factors promote tumorigenesis include the following: alteration in adiposine secretion and in related signaling pathways. Insulin-resistant hyperinsulinemia after insulin resistance and stimulation of the insulin-1-like growth factor (ILGF-1)-related axis are powerful promoters of tumor progression along with visceral adipositivity. The abundant presence of inflammatory cells in visceral adipose tissue includes macrophages and T-cells, which stimulates an inflammatory and pro-tumorigenic environment [9]. Lactation is a process corresponding to the mammary gland and is physiologically activated during pregnancy and inactivated after neonatal feeding and due to loss of suction. The post-lactation state involves an involutive homeostasis process in which apoptosis is present. The study of this process at the molecular level in animal models has demonstrated that *TIMP3* gene deficiency leads to the dysregulation of the tumor necrosis factor (TNF), to early activation of caspases, and to mitochondrial apoptosis. The first phase of involution is much accelerated and begins by the activation of proteins STAT3 and TGFβ3, together with immediate luminal destruction through the fragmentation of E-cadherin. Epithelial apoptosis is followed by accelerated adipogenesis and great infiltration of macrophages and T-cells; thus, it appears that *TIMP3* exerts an impact on apoptosis and inflammatory cell flow during the mammary involution process. An ever more precise understanding of the molecular processes of the homeostatic equilibrium in the breast is important keys in understanding carcinogenesis of the breast in pregnant women with breast cancer [10]. By means of a cell line study, the loss has been identified of Wnt signaling pathway-induced protein 3 (WISP3/CCN6; LIBC [Lost in Inflammatory Breast Cancer]). WISP3/CCN6 is a secreted protein with tumor suppressor functions that is also a member of the CCN protein family [11]. Surprisingly, CCN6 contains a binding site or "motif" similar to another of the Insulin growth factor (IGF)-like factor of IGF-binding protein-related 9 peptides (IGFBP-rp9). It is well known that high circulating levels of IGF, with the loss of IGF-binding proteins, have been associated with the risk of developing multiple tumors including breast tumors [12]. Microarray analysis in IBC compared in noninflammatory tumors has demonstrated a signature of IBC that includes genes involved in IGF signaling, which we will discuss later in the section on microarrays and genomic signatures in IBC. IGF-1 stimulates the production of inflammatory cytokines (interleukin-8 and interleukin-6) through the activation of extracellular regulatory kinases (ERK) and MAPK, which suggests that alterations in IGF-1 signaling in IBC possess important consequences in the regulation of an inflammatory microenvironment, which could be sensitive to ERK and MAPK inhibitors. Even more so, clinical and epidemiological evidence indicate an important relationship among insulin resistance, hyperinsulinemia, diabetes, and poor prognosis in patients with breast cancer. These observations are consistent with clinical observations of the existence of a significant association between body mass index (BMI) and poor prognosis in patients with locally advanced breast cancer (LABC), also including IBC [13]. At present, multiple target agents of the receptor tyrosine kinase (RTK) signaling pathway for IGF-1 have been evaluated in preclinical, and now in clinical, studies that include IGF-1 anti-receptor antibodies and small inhibitor molecules of the receptor tyrosine kinases (RTKI) for IGF-1 [14, 15]. Recent reports indicate that the administration of metformin-type antidiabetic agents results in a higher rate of complete pathological responses (CPR) to chemotherapy in patients with diabetes and breast cancer than in those who are not treated with metformin [16]. This mechanism of action of metformin includes activation of the monophosphatase adenosine-activated, energy-sensing kinase and blockade of the translation of the p70S6 kinase-1/mammal-regulated protein, which is the molecular target of rapamycin. Another mechanism demonstrated by metformin action on the tumor cell is the blockade of the activation of the phosphoinositide 3-kinase (PI3K)/Akt pathways involved in survival and proliferation, in addition to avoiding activation of the ERK [17]. All of these pathways are known to be dysregulated in breast cancer. With all of what demonstrated in the studies commented on here taken together, in addition to some others, the evidence clearly suggests that the signaling pathway, together with EGFR, ERK, MAPK, and the pro-inflammatory cytokines, could be crucial targets for the exploration of the importance of these in the regulation of aggressive IBC phenotype.

Genomic Balance in Inflammatory Breast Cancer

With respect to genomic equilibrium, important information has been published utilizing microarrays for high-resolution comparative genomic hybridization and profile expression, demonstrating that cases of IBC are heterogeneous, as are cases of noninflammatory mammary tumors. The number of altered chromosomal regions was similar in both tumor types, although some altered regions were present more frequently in IBC. Many active genes are present in both cases, although it appears that these were more commonly active in IBC. Finally, the authors present a set of 24 genes that could be markers of the disease (IBC), although it is clear that a series of statistically significant cases is necessary to validate this information. Interestingly, the 24 gene candidates are involved in protein translation, cellular cycle, RNA processing, and cell transcription, metabolism, and migration, all characteristics of a very proliferative and invasive tumor, in addition to their additionally demonstrated high genomic instability [18].

Potential Prognostic Markers in Inflammatory Breast Cancer

Overexpression of epidermal growth factor receptors (ErbB) is very common in IBC. Treatment with lapatinib-type, anti-ErbB1/2 TKI agents mediates tumor apoptosis. Cellular models of IBC have demonstrated, on the other hand, that there is an increase in the formation of reactive oxygen species (ROS), and these are blockade mechanisms of sensitivity to anti-ErbB1/2 treatment. Thus, use of antioxidants of reduction-oxidation (redox) modulators in this particular cancer type comprises negative regulators for ROS formation and accumulation [19]. On the other hand, proteins c-ErbB2, p53, Ki-67, ER, and PgR have been evaluated by immunohistochemistry in patients with IBC presenting with distant metastasis. These results only correlated with protein p53 accumulation with the presence of visceral metastases, in addition to being a predictor of poor survival [20]. In another study, the expression and correlation of the protein caveolin-1, which is a structural protein of the IBC-cell membrane caveolar microdomains (also described in breast cancer cell lines) and not in the cells of noninflammatory mammary cancer tumors was evaluated. Caveolin-1 correlated with a number of positive metastatic lymph nodes in both groups of patients. The results demonstrated that caveolin-1 is expressed in and correlates with a number of positive lymph nodes in IBC, which could explain the explosive invasive power of this mammary tumor type, and that in prospective studies with a larger number of samples, the caveolin-1 protein could be validated as a prognostic marker of lymph node metastasis in IBC [21]. A protein that has demonstrated to possess tumor suppressor properties in breast cancer is E-cadherin; likewise, it has been demonstrated that it is found to be overexpressed in IBC, allowing the formation of lymphovascular emboli, which offers cytoprotector and resistance mechanisms to the chemotherapy of IBC cells. E-cadherin activity has shown to be altered by its intracellular traffic and not by genetic overexpression mechanisms, in addition to exhibiting itself in two molecular forms, one of 120 kDa and the other of 5 kDa, which converts it into a potential marker of IBC [22]. In the murine model of the Mary-X xenoimplant, lymphovascular tumor emboli are reproduced in the skin covering the breast of the murine model, converting the mouse's skin to a brilliant red color, thus providing an adequate model with which to be able to study this phenomenon, one of the characteristic signatures of IBC. The Mary-X murine model possesses a molecular subtype present in the majority of IBC tumors: these are ER/PR/HER-2-negative but express p53 and EGFR [23]. They are characterized by the aberrant overexpression of the E-cadherin calcium-dependent transmembrane glycoprotein, which is one of the characteristics of IBC tumors and of tumor emboli, because it has also been demonstrated that E-cadherin is present on the surface of circulating tumor cells isolated from patients with IBC [24–26]. Curiously, tumor emboli of the Mary-X murine model express E-cadherin with the consequent loss of the sialyl-Lewisx/a (sLex/a) protein. A hyperactive/intact/alpha E-cadherin, beta-catenin, intervenes in the homotypical aggregation axis of cells forming tumor emboli, while the sLex/a protein is a binding mediator in tumor emboli to the endothelium through the E-selectin protein. Gain of E-cadherin and loss of sLex/a protein permits cell aggregation within tumor emboli and, at the same time, presents tumor emboli binding to the surrounding endothelium. Expression of the E-cadherin protein has been associated with a normal breast-cell phenotype, while loss of E-cadherin expression and increase of the N-cadherin protein has demonstrated that these are produced during the mesenchymal-epithelial transition (MET) and that they are associated with tumor progression and its metastasis [27]. IBC is a notable exception to the common association between loss of E-cadherin and later acquisition of a MET phenotype [24, 26]. This anomalous expression of E-cadherin in the most aggressive and metastatic of all breast cancers is provocative in light of the current idea that loss of E-cadherin is a requisite for the MET process, which is associated with acquisition of the metastatic phenotype. This can represent a unique mechanism by means of which tumor cells can possess the molecular plasticity for submitting themselves to metastatic progression or, alternatively, can represent a cell survival mechanism within tumor emboli. Some studies have already centered on E-cadherin as a potential therapeutic target and have demonstrated that E-cadherin blockade through use of anti-E-cadherin antibodies resulted in loss of the homotypical in vitro aggregation of Mary-X murine model spheroids. When these anti-E-cadherin antibodies are injected intravenously (i.v.) into Mary-X animals, the tumors with pulmonary metastasis present dissolution of the metastatic lesions. Studies in vitro with spheroids of a Mary-X murine model that contains an E-cadherin-negative dominant mutant (H-2 K [d]-E-cad) that lack the extracellular binding domain, but that conserve the D-catenin binding domain, result in loss of the homotypical aggregation. In mice, these negative dominant mutant constructions were weakly tumorigenic and did not form tumor emboli [26, 28]. Other studies utilized a SUM149 cell line to demonstrate that the presence of E-cadherin-negative dominant mutant (H-2kd-E-cad) cDNA blocks in vitro the invasion of SUM149 cells, which interestingly is associated with lesser expression of Matrix metaloproteinases (MMP), specifically enzymes MMP-1 and MMP-9. These studies suggest that the invasion and intravasion process by tumor emboli in IBC is mediated by E-cadherin and amplification of proteolytic enzymatic activity [29]. MMP are proteolytic enzymes that play an important role in the invasion and metastasis of cancer. The role of MMP is not well studied to date in IBC; however, some studies have shown that MMP 2 and 9 (MMP-2 and MMP-9) were found to be more expressed in IBC than in the noninflammatory type, which could confer a more important role on these enzymes in the progression of this type of cancer [30]. Amphiregulin (AREG) can increase the stability of the epidermal growth factor receptor (EGFR) and promote its localization in the cell membrane. Through "knockdown" models for AREG in cell cultures, it was demonstrated that the potential of SUM-149-type breast tumor cells considerably diminished the cell growth rate and its invasive or metastatic power while increasing EGFR expression [31]. AREG "knockdown" also demonstrated, by microarray analysis, modulation in the WNT and notch signaling pathways in these cells, which demonstrates that amphiregulin can be regulating the invasive phenotype of tumor cells in breast cancer and probably by EGFR activation at the cytoplasmic membrane level [31].

Genetic Expression Profiles and the Molecular Signature of the Rho C GTPase Oncogene in Inflammatory Breast Cancer

The genomic profile of IBC and of noninflammatory breast tumors stratified according to hormonal receptor state and HER2. Employing cDNA microarray technology based on the Affymetrix platform, 82 recently diagnosed mammary tumors were evaluated. Three different IBC and noninflammatory subtypes were compared: (1) ER-positive/HER2-normal, (2) HER2-amplified, and (3) ER-negative/HER2-normal; global expression results of expression were reported as follows: Pathways related with the complement and the immune system were overexpressed in ER-positive/HER2-normal IBC; similarly, protein translation and the mammalian target of rapamycin (mTOR) signaling pathway were overexpressed in HER2-amplified IBC; apoptosis and lipid- and neural metabolism-related signaling pathways were overexpressed particularly in ER-negative/HER2-normal-type IBC. The latter results demonstrate that it is possible to subclassify IBC molecularly, because there are different comparers between inflammatory and noninflammatory breast tumors [32]. One very much sought-after strategy for studying IBC has been the comparative use of the SUM149 cell line [33]. Through differential analysis of the expression between this cell line and normal lymphocytes, one of the most overregulated genes in IBC comprised the transforming *Rho C GTPase* oncogene, which codifies for a GTPase Ras (Rho)-family member that is involved in cytoskeletal reorganization during invasion as well as in the expression of pro-angiogenic factors and the production of pro-inflammatory cytokines. It has been demonstrated as overexpressed in the Rho C GTPase protein in 90 % of IBC. Interestingly, the Rho C GTPase-associated IBC phenotype is blocked by a farnesyltransferase inhibitor (FTI) [34], which has justified the study of the effect of a selective inhibitor of this enzyme-denominated tipifarnib (Zarnestra®) in a phase 2 study in patients with stage IIB–IIIC breast cancer [35]. In another study of microarrays and IBC, the differential expression was evaluated between IBC tumors and noninflammatory tumors, revealing a molecular signature that included genes involved in IGF binding and an increase in genes belonging to Rho guanyl-nucleotide exchange factor activity [5], findings consisting of gain of Rho-GTPase activity and loss of WISP3/CCN6, all as the signature of IBC.

Molecular Subtypes of Inflammatory Breast Cancer

At present, mammary tumors have already been afforded a molecular subclassification, thus providing an origin in the description of subtypes based on the presence or the absence of estrogen and progestogenic receptors (ER/PR), the claudin expression level, HER2 oncogene expression and amplification, and the differential expression of cytokeratins 5/6 and/or cytokeratins 8/18. Although IBC can possess any combination of hormonal receptors and oncogenes, these are most frequently identified within the HER2-amplified, ER/PR-negative, "basal-like," low-claudin group [36]. Another characteristic of IBC is high expression of p53 and of EGFR, which have been associated with poor prognosis [37, 38]. Determination of breast cancer molecular subtypes has principal implications for the determination of the therapeutic target that will be utilized (whether HER2 or EGFR); however, it appears that utilizing a double blockade results in greater response and efficacy in patients with IBC with HER-positive tumors, although these excellent responses in their majority do not last >12 months and generate resistance.

Toward the New Therapeutics of Inflammatory Breast Cancer: Blockade of Invasion and Metastasis Versus Latest-Generation Molecular Targets

Some studies on cell lines have already centered on blocking prostaglandin activity, in particular that of endoperoxide synthase-2, better known as cyclooxygenase-2 (COX-2), because in genetic-microarray studies on genetic expression, it has been demonstrated that COX-2 is overexpressed in IBC [39]. Overexpression of COX-2 and high levels of its product, prostaglandin E2 (PGE2), are characteristics of invasive breast tumors and are detectable at early breast cancer stages [40]. COX-2 also directly regulates the aromatase enzyme P450 Cyp191A1, by which it regulates estrogen production and interacts with HER2 as well as with EGFR. COX-2 is part of the gene group that mediates extravasation, survival, and implant at the distance of the metastasis [41]. Although nonsteroidal anti-inflammatory drugs (NSAID) such as "coxib" types are a selective class of COX-2 inhibitors, these have been promising as therapeutic and chemoprotective agents; however, their association with cardiotoxicity led to the withdrawal from the market of rofecoxib and to a reduction in the use of celecoxib. Some studies have demonstrated that antagonists of the receptor of prostanoid EP4, which blocks PGE2 binding, effectively inhibit the invasion and aberrant angiogenesis exhibited by IBC tumor cells [42]. Surprisingly, a study in the IBC of canines reported that the nonselective NSAID drug piroxicam, employed as unique agent, significantly increased progression-free global survival (GS) compared with doxorubicin-regime-based treatment [43]. It is then clear that the roles of COX-2 and that of the PGE-2-associated prostanoid receptor family are very important therapeutic targets in IBC. The presence has been demonstrated of HER2 protein, as well as of that of other EGFR-type RTK family members in different breast tumor types, already having evaluated the usefulness of erlotinib (HER1/EGFR inhibitor)-type RTKI in preclinical models in murines, in addition to a novel HER2-specific recombinant humanized antibody called pertuzumab (Omnitarg™), which blocks heterodimerization with other HER family members, in addition to another EGFR/HER2 dual inhibitor-denominated MP-412 (AV-412) [44]. It is noteworthy in preclinical research that although there are several murine models for xenoimplants in vivo, only Mary-X and WIBC-9 models recapitulate tumor emboli, which is the cytopathological signature of IBC.

References

1. Merajver SD, Sabel MS. Inflammatory breast cancer. In: Harris JR, Lippman ME, Morrow M, Osborne CK, editors. Diseases of the breast. 3rd ed. Philadelphia: Lippincott Williams and Wilkins; 2004.
2. Anderson W, Schairer C, Chen B, Hance K, Levine P. Epidemiology of inflammatory breast cancer (IBC). Breast Dis. 2005;22:9–23.
3. Hamidullah, Changkija B, Konwar R. Role of interleukin-10 in breast cancer. Breast Cancer Res Treat. 2012 May;133(1):11–21.
4. Xie G, Yao Q, Liu Y, Du S, Liu A, Guo Z, Sun A, Ruan J, Chen L, Ye C, Yuan Y. IL-6-induced epithelial-mesenchymal transition promotes the generation of breast cancer stem-like cells analogous to mammosphere cultures. Int J Oncol. 2011. doi:10.3892/ijo.2011.1275.
5. Van Laere SJ, Van der Auwera I, Van den Eynden GG, et al. NF-kappaB activation in inflammatory breast cancer is associated with oestrogen receptor down-regulation, secondary to EGFR and/or ErbB2 overexpression and MAPK hyperactivation. Br J Cancer. 2007;97:659–69.
6. Cabioglu N, Gong Y, Islam R, et al. Expression of growth factor and chemokine receptors: new insights in the biology of inflammatory breast cancer. Ann Oncol. 2007;18:1021–9.
7. Macciò A, Madeddu C. Obesity, inflammation, and postmenopausal breast cancer: therapeutic implications. Sci World J. 2011;11:2020–36. Epub 2011 Oct 27.
8. Bonafè M, Storci G, Franceschi C. Inflamm-aging of the stem cell niche: breast cancer as a paradigmatic example: breakdown of the multi-shell cytokine network fuels cancer in aged people. Bioessays. 2011. doi:10.1002/bies.201100104.
9. Doyle SL, Donohoe CL, Lysaght J, Reynolds JV. Visceral obesity, metabolic syndrome, insulin resistance and cancer. Proc Nutr Soc. 2011;3:1–9.
10. Hojilla CV, Jackson HW, Khokha R. TIMP3 regulates mammary epithelial apoptosis with immune cell recruitment through differential TNF dependence (abstract). PLoS One. 2011;6(10):e26718. Epub 2011 Oct 28.
11. Kleer CG, Zhang Y, Pan Q, Merajver SD. WISP3 (CCN6) is a secreted tumor suppressor protein that modulates IGF signaling in inflammatory breast cancer. Neoplasia. 2004;6:179–85.
12. Yu H, Rohan T. Role of the insulin-like growth factor family in cancer development and progression. J Natl Cancer Inst. 2000;92:1472–89.
13. Dawood S, Broglio K, González-Angulo AM, et al. Prognostic value of body mass index in locally advanced breast cancer. Clin Cancer Res. 2008;14:1718–25.
14. Pollak M. Targeting insulin and insulin-like growth factor signalling in oncology. Curr Opin Pharmacol. 2008;8:384–92.
15. Zha J, O'Brien C, Savage H, et al. Molecular predictors of response to a humanized antiinsulin-like

growth factor-I receptor monoclonal antibody in breast and colorectal cancer. Mol Cancer Ther. 2009; 8:2110–21.
16. Jiralerspong S, Palla SL, Giordano SH, et al. Metformin and pathologic complete responses to neoadjuvant chemotherapy in diabetic patients with breast cancer. J Clin Oncol. 2009;27:3297–302.
17. Goodwin PJ, Ligibel JA, Stambolic V. Metformin in breast cancer: time for action. J Clin Oncol. 2009; 27:3271–3.
18. Bekhouche I, Finetti P, Adelaïde J, Ferrari A, TarpinC, Charafe-Jauffret E, Charpin C, Houvenaeghel G, Jacquemier J, Bidaut G, Birnbaum D, Viens P, Chaffanet M, Bertucci F. High-resolution comparative genomic hybridization of inflammatory breast cancer and identification of candidate genes (abstract). PLoS One. 2011;6(2):e16950.
19. Aird KM, Allensworth JL, Batinic-Haberle I, Lyerly HK, Dewhirst MW, Devi GR. ErbB1/2 tyrosine kinase inhibitor mediates oxidative stress-induced apoptosis in inflammatory breast cancer cells. Breast Cancer Res Treat. 2011;132:109–19.
20. Sezgin C, Gokmen E, Kapkac M, Zekioglu O, Esassolak M, Karabulut B, Sanli UA, Uslu R. p53 protein accumulation and presence of visceral metastasis are independent prognostic factors for survival in patients with metastatic inflammatory breast carcinoma. Med Princ Pract. 2011;20(2):159–64. Epub 2011 Jan 20.
21. Nouh MA, Mohamed MM, El-Shinawi M, Shaalan MA, Cavallo-Medved D, Khaled HM, Sloane BF. Cathepsin B: a potential prognostic marker for inflammatory breast cancer (abstract). J Transl Med. 2011;9:1.
22. Ye Y, Téllez JD, Durazo M, Belcher M, Yearsley K, Barsky SH. E-cadherin accumulation within the lymphovascular embolus of inflammatory breast cancer is due to altered trafficking. Anticancer Res. 2010; 30(10):3903–10.
23. Alpaugh ML, Tomlinson JS, Shao ZM, Barsky SH. A novel human xenograft model of inflammatory breast cancer. Cancer Res. 1999;59:5079–84.
24. Kleer CG, van Golen KL, Braun T, Merajver SD. Persistent E-cadherin expression in inflammatory breast cancer. Mod Pathol. 2001;14:458–64.
25. Van den Eynden GG, Van der Auwera I, Van Laere S, et al. Validation of a tissue microarray to study differential protein expression in inflammatory and noninflammatory breast cancer. Breast Cancer Res Treat. 2004;85:13–22.
26. Tomlinson JS, Alpaugh ML, Barsky SH. An intact overexpressed E-cadherin/alpha/betacatenin axis characterizes the lymphovascular emboli of inflammatory breast carcinoma. Cancer Res. 2001;61:5231–41.
27. Kalluri R, Weinberg RA. The basics of epithelial-mesenchymal transition. J Clin Invest. 2009;119:1420–8.
28. Alpaugh ML, Barsky SH. Reversible model of spheroid formation allows for high efficiency of gene delivery *ex vivo* and accurate gene assessment *in vivo*. Hum Gene Ther. 2002;13:1245–58.
29. Dong HM, Liu G, Hou YF, et al. Dominant-negative E-cadherin inhibits the invasiveness of inflammatory breast cancer cells in vitro. J Cancer Res Clin Oncol. 2007;133:83–92.
30. Al-Raawi D, Abu-El-Zahab H, El-Shinawi M, Mohamed MM. Membrane type-1 matrix metalloproteinase (MT1-MMP) correlates with the expression and activation of matrix metalloproteinase-2 (MMP-2) in inflammatory breast cancer. Int J Clin Exp Med. 2011;4(4):265–75. Epub 2011 Oct 11.
31. Baillo A, Giroux C, Ethier SP. Knock-down of amphiregulin inhibits cellular invasion in inflammatory breast cancer. J Cell Physiol. 2011;226(10):2691–701. doi:10.1002/jcp. 22620.
32. Iwamoto T, Bianchini G, Qi Y, Cristofanilli M, Lucci A, Woodward WA, Reuben JM, Matsuoka J, Gong Y, Krishnamurthy S, Valero V, Hortobagyi GN, Robertson F, Symmans WF, Pusztai L, Ueno NT. Different gene expressions are associated with the different molecular subtypes of inflammatory breast cancer. Breast Cancer Res Treat. 2011;125(3): 785–95. Epub 2010 Dec 9.
33. Forozan F, Veldman R, Ammerman CA, et al. Molecular cytogenetic analysis of 11 new breast cancer cell lines. Br J Cancer. 1999;81: 1328–34.
34. van Golen KL, Bao L, DiVito MM, Wu Z, Prendergast GC, Merajver SD. Reversion of RhoC GTPase-induced inflammatory breast cancer phenotype by treatment with a farnesyl transferase inhibitor. Mol Cancer Ther. 2002;1:575–83.
35. Sparano JA, Moulder S, Kazi A, et al. Phase II trial of tipifarnib plus neoadjuvant doxorubicin-cyclophosphamide in patients with clinical stage IIB-IIIC breast cancer. Clin Cancer Res. 2009;15:2942–8.
36. Van Laere SJ, Van den Eynden GG, Van der Auwera I, et al. Identification of cell-of-origin breast tumor subtypes in inflammatory breast cancer by gene expression profiling. Breast Cancer Res Treat. 2006;95:243–55.
37. González-Angulo AM, Sneige N, Buzdar AU, et al. p53 expression as a prognostic marker in inflammatory breast cancer. Clin Cancer Res. 2004;10:6215–21.
38. Guerin M, Gabillot M, Mathieu MC, et al. Structure and expression of *c-erbB-2* and *EGF* receptor genes in inflammatory and non-inflammatory breast cancer: prognostic significance. Int J Cancer. 1989;43:201–8.
39. Van der Auwera I, Van Laere SJ, Van den Eynden GG, et al. Increased angiogenesis and lymphangiogenesis in inflammatory versus noninflammatory breast cancer by real-time reverse transcriptase-PCR gene expression quantification. Clin Cancer Res. 2004;10:7965–71.
40. Parrett ML, Harris RE, Joarder FS, Ross MS, Clausen KP, Robertson FM. Cyclooxygenase-2 gene expression in human breast cancer. Int J Oncol. 1997; 10:503–7.
41. Nguyen DX, Bos PD, Massague J. Metastasis: from dissemination to organ-specific colonization. Nat Rev Cancer. 2009;9:274–84.

42. Robertson FM, Simeone AM, Mazumdar A, et al. Molecular and pharmacological blockade of the EP4 receptor selectively inhibits both proliferation and invasion of human inflammatory breast cancer cells. J Exp Ther Oncol. 2008;7:299–312.
43. de Souza CH M, Toledo-Piza E, Amorin R, Barboza A, Tobias KM. Inflammatory mammary carcinoma in 12 dogs: clinical features, cyclooxygenase-2 expression, and response to piroxicam treatment. Can Vet J. 2009;50:506–10.
44. Suzuki T, Fujii A, Ohya J, et al. Antitumor activity of a dual epidermal growth factor receptor and ErbB2 kinase inhibitor MP-412 (AV-412) in mouse xenograft models. Cancer Sci. 2009;100:1526–31.

Target Therapy in Inflammatory Breast Cancer

10

Flavia Morales-Vasquez, Horacio Noe Lopez-Basave, Claudia Arce-Salinas, Jose Luis Aguilar-Ponce, and Oscar Gerardo Arrieta-Rodriguez

Target Therapy

Despite that this entity in oncology is a very good demonstration of what can be offered by multimodal treatment in cancer, providing the best opportunities for the patient, the prognosis of inflammatory breast cancer (IBC) is poor.

Systemic treatment with chemotherapy (CT) and other target therapies appears today to be the cornerstone in the management of this disease.

Treatment of IBC usually initiates with neoadjuvant CT because prior to offering surgical management, the problem of infiltration into the skin should be resolved.

F. Morales-Vasquez, M.D., M.S. (✉)
C. Arce-Salinas, M.D., M.Sc.
Department of Medical Oncology, Instituto Nacional de Cancerologia-Mexico, San Fernando Num 22, Tlalpan, Mexico City, DF 14080, Mexico
e-mail: fabymvmizpah@aol.com

H.N. Lopez-Basave, M.S.
Department of Oncological Surgery, Instituto Nacional de Cancerologia-Mexico, Mexico City, DF, Mexico

J.L. Aguilar-Ponce, M.D.
Department of Medical Oncology, Instituto Nacional de Cancerologia-Mexico, San Fernando Num 22, Tlalpan, Mexico City, DF 14080, Mexico

O.G. Arrieta-Rodriguez, M.D.
Department of Medical Oncology, Instituto Nacional de Cancerologia-Mexico, Mexico City, DF, Mexico

The selection and order of CT drugs will be carried out based on the patient's characteristics, the tumor type in terms of its histological component, the grade and histological and molecular markers that it expresses, the disease extension, and the options and resources available. The type of CT agent or the scheme selected and the exact number of cycles will depend on the clinical evolution. At present, there is no standard treatment, and the tendency is toward the design of treatments that are appropriate for the characteristics of each case.

Several distinctive biological characterize and separate IBC from noninflammatory breast cancer. These are characteristics that are associated with poor prognosis and include a high S-phase fraction, high grade, aneuploidy, loss of hormonal receptors, and overexpression of human epithelial receptor-2 (HER2) [1, 2]. Inflammatory carcinomas more frequently present in p-53-level mutations, which is related with tumor progression, diminution in response to CT, and reduction in the results of global survival (GS) [3]. Inflammatory carcinoma tumors of the breast overexpress E-cadherin, a calcium-regulating transmembrane glycoprotein that promotes cell-cell adhesion and through this, promotes invasion with tumor emboli of the dermal lymphatic system [4]. The dysregulation of p27kip1, a cyclin-dependent kinase (CDK) implicated in the inhibition of apoptosis, cellular adhesion, the promotion of cellular differentiation, and regulation of drug resistance [5], in addition to the widely known characteristics of microvasculature increase, high endothelial-cell proliferation,

J.G. de la Garza-Salazar et al. (eds.), *Inflammatory Breast Cancer*,
DOI 10.1007/978-0-85729-991-8_10, © Springer-Verlag London 2013

and the expression of lymphangiogenetic factors (VEGF-C, VEGF-D, VEGFR-3, Prox-1), and the lymphatic vascular endothelial receptor 1 and angiogenic factors (Basic fibroblast growth factor [bFGF], Vascular endothelial growth factor [VEGF], Interleukin-6 [IL-6], and IL-8) [6, 7].

Several genes have been identified that contribute to the aggressive behavior of IBC, such as those related with the nuclear factor-kappa beta (NF-kB) [8], this being an important mediator of migration, invasion, and development of metastasis. The differential expression of other genes [9] has also been reported as overexpression of RboC guanosine triphosphatase (GTPase) and loss of WNT-1 induced by the secreted protein 3 (*WISP3*). The role of these genes has been studied because they contribute to the metastatic potential of IBC in overregulating angiogenic factors (VEGF and bFGF) and in promoting the motility and invasion and disruption of cell bonds.

WISP3 is a tumor suppressor gene that codifies the insulin-like growth factor-related protein that regulates tumor cell growth, invasion, and angiogenesis [9]. Loss of *WISP3* expression contributes to the aggressive IBC phenotype.

The advent of new biological treatments has represented an additional benefit because the percentages of pathological response (PR) have improved and there is even better prognosis. Among the molecular differences that are decisive in IBC, we find HER1 and HER2 overexpression. However, given the reduced frequency of this entity, there is at present no adequate biomolecular characterization of it. Precisely, it remains unknown whether the proportion of patients with the HER2-positive subtype, or with the basal-like subtype, is greater than those with the A and B luminal subtypes, as we suppose.

Trastuzumab and lapatinib, agents directed against HER2, have demonstrated an indubitable clinical benefit in the population of patients with breast cancer who overexpress HER2. The Wnt1-pathway protein 3 inducer; the homologous gene *Ras*, a member of the guanosine-triphosphatase family; the epidermal growth factor receptor (EGFR); and the protein p27 (kip1) have also been studied as potential therapeutic targets in IBC. On the other hand, molecular targets in the vasculolymphatic process (angiogenesis, lymphangiogenesis, and vasculogenesis) have demonstrated enormous potential. Although the loss of E-cadherin is an indicator that there is a mesenchymal-epithelial transition (MET) and that this could be related with a greater tendency toward the promotion of metastatic activity, paradoxically, overexpression of E-cadherin in IBC is carried out by means of an unknown molecular mechanism.

The systematic management of IBC has evolved interestingly over the past four decades. IBC has always been considered a disease with a fatal evolution, and even in the 1960s, patients with IBC were treated with surgery and radiotherapy (RT); thus, 5-year survival rates of only 5 % were reported, with a median survival of 2.4–5 months [10]. In Mexico, De la Garza and collaborators initiated, from the 1970s, multimodal management for this group of patients, with improvements in global survival (GS) [11]. Ueno and colleagues [12] reported in 1997 at MD Anderson Cancer Center (MDACC) series of patients treated with CT based on 5-fluorouracil (5-FU), adriamycin, and cyclophosphamide (FAC) plus RT with or without surgery and reported 5-year survival indices of 40 %. In the most recent decade with the incorporation of target therapies, reports cite an improvement in the 4-year survival rate of 86 % in a very small series of cases treated with CT that combined anthracyclines, taxanes, and platinum plus trastuzumab, reported by Hurley et al. [13]. These findings confirm the potential of target therapy.

Therapy Directed Against HER2

Approximately of breast cancer tumors show a 25 % overexpression of HER2. Some publications suggest that overexpression is greater in IBC, but there are no decisive numbers. However, HER2 overexpression undoubtedly correlates with a more aggressive phenotype and poorer prognostic results [14]. HER2 (also known as ErbB2) is a member of the tyrosine-kinase receptor (TKR) family of the epidermal growth factor

(EGF); in humans, four members are described: HER1, HER2, HER3, and HER4. Each is a transmembrane receptor with partial homology that normally regulates cell growth and survival, adhesion, migration, and differentiation, as well as other cellular responses [15]. Each receptor is constituted of an extracellular binding domain, a transmembrane lipophilic segment, and (with the exception of HER3) a functional intracellular TK domain. TK domains are activated as much by homo- as by heterodimerization, which are generally induced by binding with the ligand, although to date no natural ligand for HER2 has been identified. Dimerization in the absence of a ligand can take place when the HER2 extracellular domain adopts a fixed configuration comprising a ligand-activation-like state [16] and by overexpression and mutation of the receptor. Once activated, the transduction cascades of the signals of these receptors promote cellular proliferation through the (Ras-mitogen-activated protein kinase [MAPK]) pathway, as well as survival through inhibition of programmed cellular death through the phosphatidylinositol 3-kinase/Akt objective of the mammalian target of rapamycin (mTOR) pathway [17]. Clinically, overexpression is detected by immunohistochemistry, with an antibody directed against the HER2 receptor, or by means of fluorescence in situ hybridization (FISH), which utilizes a DNA fluorescence-marked catheter on the *ERBB2* gene with the purpose of detecting the number of gene copies.

Trastuzumab

There are target therapy options for HER2 as well as for HER1 TK family members. The monoclonal antibody trastuzumab directed against the HER2 protein has demonstrated improvement in GS for early-stage breast cancer as well as for advanced or metastatic breast cancer [18–20]. Some authors, such as Buzdar et al. [21] and Dawood et al. [22], combined this target therapy with CT schemes that contained anthracyclines and taxanes; the former author with operable breast cancer; and the latter, in patients with advanced breast cancer (which included IBC), demonstrating better percentages of pathological response (PR).

While several studies report that in IBC, greater HER2 overexpression is observed, which makes trastuzumab, a monoclonal antibody, an ideal agent to add to the treatment of patients with IBC who overexpress HER2, several authors have proposed studies in which some CT schemes are combined with this monoclonal antibody.

Hurley and colleagues [13] reported on a cohort of 48 patients with locally advanced breast cancer (LABC) (including IBC) who were treated for 12 weeks with docetaxel, cisplatin, and trastuzumab followed by surgery, adjuvant CT, and RT. In the study, PR was reported in 17 %. Van Pelt et al. [23] reported a 22-patient cohort (nine with IBC) with patients treated with docetaxel and trastuzumab and in which a 40 % response was observed. Limentani and colleagues [24] indicated treatment with docetaxel, Navelbine, and trastuzumab in 31 patients with clinical response in 94 % and PR in 39 %. Burstein et al. [25] in a pilot study of 40 patients with clinical stages II and III that included IBC, reported the following responses: clinical response in 30 % and PR in 18 %. Without doubt, the evidence shows that trastuzumab is a useful agent in patients with IBC who overexpress HER2; however, defining an even better combination scheme or the ideal sequence remains to be found for obtaining better results.

Lapatinib

Lapatinib (Tykerb, GlaxoSmithKline) is a reversible inhibitor of ErbB1 and ErbB2 that has shown, in ErbB1/ErbB2-expressing cell lines, to induce cellular arrest and apoptosis. Geyer and colleagues [26] reported a cohort of patients who were HER2-positive with LABC or metastatic breast cancer who had been treated with CT plus trastuzumab and with progressive disease, who were randomized to receive capecitabine alone versus capecitabine plus lapatinib. The authors found that the combination that included lapatinib reduced the risk of disease progression in 51 %. Partial responses were observed in patients with IBC who were multitreated. Based on observation of the usefulness of these biological agents, Cristofanilli and colleagues evaluated the combination of lapatinib and paclitaxel in 21 patients with HER2 overexpression and IBC, observing clinical responses of 95 %; thus, these results are being validated in prospective clinical assays [27].

Among the advantages of lapatinib, we have that although it is more toxic at the gastrointestinal level (diarrhea and nausea), at the dermatological level (exanthema), and fatigue, it is generally well tolerated, with less cardiotoxicity [28], and better central nervous system (CNS) penetration.

Based on preclinical findings that indicate synergic activity between lapatinib and trastuzumab and an absence of cross-resistance [29], this combination is being studied in clinical assays. A phase III study was reported with 296 patients with trastuzumab-refractory multitreated metastatic breast cancer who were randomized to lapatinib against lapatinib-trastuzumab. The combined-therapy treatment arm showed greater progression-free survival (PFS): 12 versus 8.4 weeks; HR, 0.77; 95 % confidence interval (95 % CI), 0.6–1.0; and $p=0.029$ in comparison with the monotherapy. Likewise, toxicity was in general terms greater, although acceptable, for the combination [30].

Other Therapies Directed Against HER2

Pertuzumab

Pertuzumab is a humanized monoclonal antibody directed against the extracellular domain of HER2 receptor dimerization and acts by obstructing the dimerization. The different and partially complementary mechanism of action is the theoretical basis for combining pertuzumab and trastuzumab. A phase II study that approached HER2-positive, trastuzamub-refractory, metastatic breast cancer demonstrated an objective response rate (ORR) of 33 %. Therefore, this study is currently found in the course of a phase III study, the Clinical Evaluation of Pertuzumab and Trastuzumab (CLEOPATRA) study [31].

Neratinib

Neratinib is an orally reversible HER1 and 2 (tyrosine-kinase inhibitor (TKI)). Phase I preliminary data demonstrate partial response. Some small phase II studies showed this benefit: response rate, 27 % (95 % CI, 13–46 %) plus an increase in PFS of 19 weeks (95 % CI, 13–46 %) [32]; thus, these are currently found in the course of some phase III studies in metastatic breast cancer and an extended adjuvancy study after trastuzumab.

Tratuzumab-DM1

Trastuzumab-DM1 (T-DM1) is a conjugated antibody agent that utilizes trastuzumab to transport the antimicrotubular agent DM1. The hypothesis that sustains this conjugated agent is that after binding to HER2, T-MD1 undergoes receptor-mediated internalization with the intracellular release of DM1, which favors directed cell destruction with low toxicity. A phase I study demonstrated clinical activity with a maximum tolerated dose (MTD) of 3.6 mg/kg; the clinical benefit index was reported in 73 %. Reported toxicities describe transaminasemia, thrombocytopenia, and fatigue; cardiac toxicity was not cited [33]. A phase II study with 112 patients previously treated with a median of three schemes of CT and progression to a previous anti-HER2 therapy reported an ORR of 39.2 % at 4.6 months. The most frequent G 3–4 adverse event was thrombocytopenia (7.1 %) [34], confirming its activity in multitreated tumors with an acceptable toxicity, which sustains the development of phase III studies, such as the EMILIA/TDM4370g study, which compares T-DM1 versus capecitabine plus lapatinib in patients previously treated with trastuzumab.

mTOR Inhibitors

The serine/threonine kinase mTOR is a cascade component under the PTEN/PI3K pathway. The mTOR pathway performs a central role in the regulation of cell growth, proliferation, and survival. In addition, as previously analyzed, loss of PTEN expression and/or activation of PI3K/Akt protein signaling transducers can be possible mechanisms of resistance to trastuzumab. Two mTOR inhibitors, temsinolimus and everolimus, are found in the developmental stage, with everolimus the most promising agent. In preclinical and clinical estudies, this two mTOR inhibitors, there was inhibition of tumor growth in cells previously challenged with trastuzumab and in tumors also previously exposed to trastuzumab, evidencing that resistance to trastuzumab can be overcome [35]. The limiting toxicities of the most frequently administered doses were neutropenia and stomatitis. Efficiency has been constant in the combination with paclitaxel and vinorelbine [36, 37].

Due to favorable results in phase I and II studies, we find phase III studies that are currently evaluating everolimus in a combination of CT with trastuzumab, that is, the Breast Cancer Trials of Oral Everolimus (BOLERO)-1 and BOLERO-3 studies.

Temsirolimus, the other mTOR inhibitor, although when its synergic effect was tested on combining it with hormonal therapy, a phase III study in combination with letrozole as first-line treatment in metastatic disease, was closed prematurely after a planned intermediate analysis due to lack of efficacy [38].

Antiangiogenic Therapy

Angiogenesis is recognized as a fundamental process in the progression and the development of metastasis in cancer. Specially in breast cancer, the majority of tumors express multiple angiogenic factors, and, as previously explained, we precisely find the following in IBC: an important increase in microvasculature, high endothelial proliferation, and the expression of lymphangiogenetic factors (VEGF-C, VEGF-D, VEGFR-3, Prox-1, the lymphatic vascular endothelial vascular receptor 1 and angiogenetic factors (including bFGF, VEGF, interleukin-6 (IL-6), and IL-8)) [6, 7].

VEGF presents a diversity of isoforms; however, the functioning of the diverse isoforms is not well defined, but it is known that VEGF-A is the isoform that induces vasodilation and pathological angiogenesis with greatest potency. In breast cancer, high levels have been detected of the messenger RNA (mRNA) of VEGF, and it has been demonstrated that this characteristic is associated with worse disease-free survival (DFS) rates and less GS [39].

Given that IBC is a disease that is characterized by its high vascularity, McCarthy et al. evaluated microvascular density (MVD) by immunohistochemistry in 67 breast cancer tumors of women from Tunis, Tunisia, with or without the inflammatory cancer phenotype; the intratumor microvascular count was 25.5 in IBC against 6.5 in noninflammatory breast cancer [40].

For this characteristic, VEGF blockage purports to reduce the tumor vascularity number in order to reduce the number of circulating endothelial and progenitor cells, especially in IBC; to increase disease control; and to reduce the metastatic potential.

Among agents found currently under study for the treatment of IBC, such as treatments directed against angiogenic factors, bevacizumab is highlighted. Bevacizumab is a humanized monoclonal antibody against all VEGF-A isoforms. It has been evaluated in diverse clinical studies in the metastatic ambit in combination with CT but has shown limited efficacy. The first study that reported its use in combination with capecitabine in patients who had been previously treated with anthracyclines and taxanes demonstrated an increase in ORR (19.8 vs. 9.1 %), but bevacizumab did not improve PFS (4.9 vs. 4.2 months, $HR = 0.98$, $p = 0.857$) [41].

The Eastern Cooperative Oncology Group (ECOG), in the E2100 study, evaluated the use of bevacizumab and paclitaxel against paclitaxel alone in first-line treatment in metastatic breast cancer. The combination showed an increase in PFS and in the GS index, without exerting an impact on the improvement of GS: 11 versus 6 months, $p \leq 0.001$, and 28 versus 14 %, respectively [42].

In the National Cancer Institute (NCI)-0173 study, in a pilot assay of 21 patients with IBC and previously treated LABC, administration was proposed of an initial cycle of bevacizumab, followed by eight cycles of doxorubicin and docetaxel every 21 days. After locoregional control, eight cycles were offered of bevacizumab with or without hormonal treatment, according to whether the latter was indicated or not.

The objective of the study was to evaluate the molecular changes observed in the VEGF, activation of the phosphorylated VEGF2 receptor (VEGFR2), total VEGFR2, tumor microvessel density (MVD), apoptosis, and proliferation. The authors employed dynamic contrast-enhanced nuclear magnetic resonance (NMR) to evaluate vascular permeability. They observed a partial clinical response of 67 %, stable disease of 24 %, and progressive disease in 9 %. One patient presented complete PR. Global response (GR) was 67 % (95 % CI, 43–85.4 %) [43].

The 67 % GR reported in the NCI-0173 study with patients who presented IBC and LABC treated with neoadjuvant bevacizumab alone or with CT was encouraging. A decline of 66.7 % was additionally reported in phosphorylated VEGFR2 in tumor cells ($p=0.004$), and an increase of 128.8 % in apoptosis ($p=0.0008$), after one cycle of bevacizumab alone, this is observed in a CT-like manner [43]. This suggests that VEGF blockage inhibits VEGFR2 activation and induced apoptosis. However, the molecular markers that can predict treatment response are not yet fully understood. In this and other studies, attempts have been made to identify biomarkers as well as a genetic signature that permits distinguishing patients who will have a response from those who will not respond to any treatment. Thus, the authors measured CD31, an endothelial adhesion molecule, and PDGFR-b, a VEGF-A receptor, both tumor angiogenesis markers, in basal fashion, after bevacizumab alone and also after bevacizumab with CT. CD31 and the platelet-derived growth factor receptor (PDGFR)-b were expressed significantly in those who responded to treatment versus. those who did not: median of 33.5 versus 0.25; $p=0.0004$ and median of 5.9 versus 0.6; $p=0.01$, respectively. Tumor VEGF-A, now known as the bevacizumab target, was greater at baseline and exhibited a tendency to be associated with response to the entire treatment. Other biomarkers, such as microvascular density (MVD), Ki67, p53, and apoptosis, were not associated with the response.

Of the 1,339 genes selected, 26 were expressed in a way that was very different between responders and nonresponders ($p < 0.005$). The genes were classified to determine VEGFR activity, and mitosis were significantly associated with response to bevacizumab followed by bevacizumab plus CT. Therefore, the greater the tumor genetic expression of VEGFA, CD31, and PDGFR-b, the greater the treatment benefit of bevacizumab plus CT, which suggests that bevacizumab can become an agent of target therapy, although these findings remain under confirmation in another clinical assay with a larger cohort of patients.

TKI of the VEGF Receptor

SU5416 (semaxanib), a small organic molecule that inhibits VEGF-mediated signaling through a tyrosine kinase (Flk-1/KDR) (VEGFR2), was combined with doxorubicin in a phase IB study with patients with stages IIIB or IV and IBC [44]. Eighteen patients participated in this clinical assay. Neutropenia was the limiting dose and GS was not explored. Congestive heart failure presented in four (22 %) patients, which prohibited further investigation of SU5416 with doxorubicin. There was an important decrease in tumor blood flow and a trend toward diminution of MVD after treatment. Currently, some multitarget tyrosine-kinase inhibitors and other farnesyltransferase inhibitors in combination with CT in IBC are under study [45, 46]. A phase III, randomized multicenter study compared the combination of pazopanib and lapatinib against lapatinib as monotherapy in patients with IBC who overexpressed HER2 is underway at present. There also is an open-treatment arm of pazopanib for designation between pazopanib or lapatinib as monotherapy considering more safety for the patient with IBC. Pazopanib is an angiogenesis inhibitor that selectively inhibits the following: VEGFR, PDGFR, and c-kit, which are very important proteins involved in angiogenesis. For study eligibility, requirements include having presented progression to previous treatment with CT and trastuzumab. The primary objective is to evaluate PFS, while secondary objectives include GS, global response, safety, and tolerability. There are several clinical assays found that are now evaluating CT regimens in combination with target therapies for adequate management of IBC.

Conclusions

At present, a standard systemic treatment has yet not been defined for this particular pathology nor has the most appropriate sequence been found for the application of CT, target therapy, or RT, but now there are new therapeutic resources, and progress is being made toward new horizons in the management of inflammatory breast cancer (IBC).

References

1. Kleer CG, van Golen KL, Merajver SD. Molecular biology of breast cancer metastases inflammatory breast cancer: clinical syndrome and molecular determinants. Breast Cancer Res. 2000;2:423–9.
2. Turpin E, Bieche I, Berthaeau P, et al. The increased incidence of ERBB2 over expression and *TP53* mutation in inflammatory breast cancer. Oncogene. 2002;21: 7593–7.
3. González-Angulo AM, Sneige N, Kau SW, et al. p53 expression as a prognostic marker in inflammatory breast cancer. Clin Cancer Res. 2004;10:6215–21.
4. Tomlinson JS, Aplaugh ML, Barsky SH. An intact overexpressed E-cadherin/alpha, beta-catenin axis characterizes the lymphovascular emboli of inflammatory breast carcinoma. Cancer Res. 2001; 61:5231–41.
5. González-Angulo AM, Guarneri V, Gong Y, et al. Down-regulation of the cyclin-dependent kinase inhibitor p27kip1 might correlate with poor disease-free and over-all survival in inflammatory breast cancer. Clin Breast Cancer. 2006;7:326–30.
6. Van der Auwera I, Van Laere SJ, Van Den Eyden GG, et al. Increased angiogenesis and lymphagiogenesis in inflammatory versus noninflammatory breast cancer by real-time reverse transcriptase-PCR gene expression quantification. Clin Cancer Res. 2004;10: 7965–71.
7. Van der Auwera I, Van Den Eyden GG, Copaert CG, et al. Tumor lymphangiogenesis in inflammatory breast carcinoma: a histomorphometric study. Clin Cancer Res. 2005;11:7637–42.
8. Van Laere SJ, Van Den Eyden GG, Van der Auwera I, et al. Identification of cell-of origin breast tumor subtypes in inflammatory breast cancer by gene expression profiling. Breast Cancer Res Treat. 2006;95: 243–55.
9. Van Golen KL, Davies S, Wu ZF, et al. A novel putative low-affinity insulin-like growth factor-binding protein LIBC (lost in inflammatory breast cancer) and RhoC GTPase correlate with the inflammatory breast cancer phenotype. Clin Cancer Res. 1995;5: 2511–9.
10. Bossetti F, Saccozzi R, Lena MD, Salvadori B. Inflammatory cancer of the breast: analysis of 114 cases. J Surg Oncol. 1981;18:355–61.
11. De la Garza JG, De la Huerta R, Torres TR, Sánchez BC. Different management of inflammatory breast carcinoma. Experience in 18 cases, during a period of 6 years (1970–76). In: Proceedings of the Annual American Society of Clinical Oncology, Denver, 1977 (Abstract no. C-32).
12. Ueno NT, Buzdar AU, Singletary SE, et al. Combined modality treatment of inflammatory breast carcinoma: twenty years of experience at MD Anderson Cancer Center. Cancer Chemother Pharmacol. 1997;40: 321–9.
13. Hurley J, Doliny P, Reis I, et al. Docetaxel, cisplatin, and trastuzumab as primary systemic therapy for human epidermal growth factor receptor 2-positive locally advanced breast cancer. J Clin Oncol. 2006; 24:1831–8.
14. Slamon DJ, Clark GM, Wong SG, et al. Human breast cancer correlation of relapse and survival with amplification of the HER-2/neu oncogene. Science. 1987;235:177–82.
15. Yarden Y. The EGFR family and its ligands in human cancer signaling mechanisms and therapeutic opportunities. Eur J Cancer. 2001;37 Suppl 4:S3–8.
16. Cho HS, Mason K, Ramyar KX, et al. Structure of the extracellular region of HER2 alone and in complex with the Herceptin Fab. Nature. 2003;421:756–60.
17. Yarden Y, Sliwkowski MX. Untangling the ErbB signaling network. Nat Rev Mol Cell Biol. 2001;2: 127–37.
18. Piccart-Gebhart MJ, Procter M, Leyland-Jones B, et al. Trastuzumab after adjuvant chemotherapy in HER2-positive breast cancer. N Engl J Med. 2005; 353:1659–84.
19. Romond EH, Pérez EA, Bryant J, et al. Trastuzumab plus adjuvant chemotherapy in HER2-positive breast cancer. N Engl J Med. 2005;353:1673–84.
20. Slamon DJ, Leyland-Jones B, Shak S, et al. Human breast cancer: use of chemotherapy plus a monoclonal antibody against HER2 for metastatic breast cancer that overexpress HER2. N Engl J Med. 2001;344: 783–92.
21. Buzdar AU, Ibrahim NK, Francis D, et al. Significantly higher pathologic complete remission rate after neoadjuvant therapy with trastuzumab, paclitaxel, and epirubicin chemotherapy: results of a randomized trial in human epidermal growth

receptor 2-positive operable breast cancer. J Clin Oncol. 2005;23:3676–85.
22. Dawood S, González-Angulo AM, Peintinger F, et al. Efficacy and safety of neoadjuvant trastuzumab combined with paclitaxel and epirubicin: a retrospective review of the MD Anderson experience. Cancer. 2007;110:1195–200.
23. Van Pelt AE, Mohsin S, Elledge RM, et al. Neoadjuvant trastuzumab and docetaxel in breast cancer: preliminary results. Clin Breast Cancer. 2003;4:348–53.
24. Limentani SA, Brufsky AM, Erban JK, et al. Phase II study of neoadjuvant docetaxel, vinorelbine, and trastuzumab followed by surgery and adjuvant doxorubicin plus cyclophosphamide in women with human epidermal growth factor receptor 2-overexpressing locally advanced breast cancer. J Clin Oncol. 2007;25:1232–8.
25. Burstein HJ, Harris LN, Gelman R, et al. Preoperative therapy with trastuzumab and paclitaxel followed by sequential adjuvant doxorubicin/cyclophosphamide for HER2 overexpressing stage II or III breast cancer: a pilot study. J Clin Oncol. 2003;21:46–53.
26. Geyer CE, Foster J, Lindquist D, et al. Lapatinib plus Capecitabine for HER2-positive advanced breast cancer. N Engl J Med. 2006;355:2733–43.
27. Cristofanilli M, Boussen H, Baselga J, et al. A phase II combination study of lapatinib and paclitaxel as a neo-adjuvant therapy in patients with newly diagnosed inflammatory breast cancer (IBC). Breast Cancer Res Treat. 2006;100(Suppl I):S5. Abstr1.
28. Pérez EA, Koehler M, Byrne J, et al. Cardiac safety of lapatinib: pooled analysis of 3689 patients enrolled in clinical trials. Mayo Clin Proc. 2008;83:679–86.
29. Konecny GE, Pegram MD, Venkatesan N, et al. Activity of the dual kinase inhibitor lapatinib (GW572016) against HER-2-overexpressing and trastuzumab-treated breast cancer cells. Cancer Res. 2006;66:1630–9.
30. Wu Y, Amonkar MM, Sherrill BH, O'Shaughnessy J, Ellis C, Baselga J, Blackwell KL, Burstein HJ. Impact of lapatinib plus trastuzumab versus single-agent lapatinib on quality of life of patients with trastuzumab-refractory HER2+ metastatic breast cancer. Ann Oncol. 2011;22:2582–90.
31. Baselga J, Gelmon KA, Verma S, Wardley A, Conte P, Miles D, Bianchi G, Cortes J, McNally VA, Ross GA, Fumoleau P, Gianni L. Phase II trial of pertuzumab and trastuzumab in patients with human epidermal growth factor receptor 2-positive metastatic breast cancer that progressed during prior trastuzumab therapy. J Clin Oncol. 2010;28(7):1138–44. Epub 2010 Feb 1.
32. Wong KK, Fracasso PM, Bukowski RM, Lynch TJ, Munster PN, Shapiro GI, Jänne PA, Eder JP, Naughton MJ, Ellis MJ, Jones SF, Mekhail T, Zacharchuk C, Vermette J, Abbas R, Quinn S, Powell C, Burris HA. A phase I study with neratinib (HKI-272), an irreversible pan ErbB receptor tyrosine kinase inhibitor, in patients with solid tumors. Clin Cancer Res. 2009;15(7):2552–8. Epub 2009 Mar 24.
33. Krop IE, Beeram M, Modi S, Jones SF, Holden SN, Yu W, Girish S, Tibbitts J, Yi JH, Sliwkowski MX, Jacobson F, Lutzker SG, Burris HA. Phase I study of trastuzumab-DM1, an HER2 antibody-drug conjugate, given every 3 weeks to patients with HER2-positive metastatic breast cancer. J Clin Oncol. 2010;28(16):2698–704. Epub 2010 Apr 26.
34. Burris 3rd HA, Rugo HS, Vukelja SJ, Vogel CL, Borson RA, Limentani S, Tan-Chiu E, Krop IE, Michaelson RA, Girish S, Amler L, Zheng M, Chu YW, Klencke B, O'Shaughnessy JA. Phase II study of the antibody drug conjugate trastuzumab-DM1 for the treatment of human epidermal growth factor receptor 2 (HER2)-positive breast cancer after prior HER2-directed therapy. J Clin Oncol. 2011;29(4):398–405. Epub 2010 Dec 20.
35. Morrow PK, Wulf GM, Ensor J, Booser DJ, Moore JA, Flores PR, Xiong Y, Zhang S, Krop IE, Winer EP, Kindelberger DW, Coviello J, Sahin AA, Núñez R, Hortobagyi GN, Yu D, Esteva FJ. Phase I/II study of trastuzumab in combination with everolimus (RAD001) in patients with HER2-overexpressing metastatic breast cancer who progressed on trastuzumab-based therapy. J Clin Oncol. 2011;29(23):3126–32. Epub 2011 Jul 5.
36. Jerusalem G, Fasolo A, Dieras V, Cardoso F, Bergh J, Vittori L, Zhang Y, Massacesi C, Sahmoud T, Gianni L. Phase I trial of oral mTOR inhibitor everolimus in combination with trastuzumab and vinorelbine in pre-treated patients with HER2-overexpressing metastatic breast cancer. Breast Cancer Res Treat. 2011;125(2):447–55. Epub 2010 Nov 25.
37. Andre F, Campone M, O'Regan R, Manlius C, Massacesi C, Sahmoud T, Mukhopadhyay P, Soria JC, Naughton M, Hurvitz SA. Phase I study of everolimus plus weekly paclitaxel and trastuzumab in patients with metastatic breast cancer pretreated with trastuzumab. J Clin Oncol. 2010;28(34):5110–5. Epub 2010 Oct 25.
38. Chan S, Scheulen ME, Johnston S, Mross K, Cardoso F, Dittrich C, Eiermann W, Hess D, Morant R, Semiglazov V, Borner M, Salzberg M, Ostapenko V, Illiger HJ, Behringer D, Bardy-Bouxin N, Boni J, Kong S, Cincotta M, Moore L. Phase II study of temsinolimus (CCI-779), a novel inhibitor of mTOR, in heavily pretreated patients with locally advanced or metastatic breast cancer. J Clin Oncol. 2005;23(23):5314–22. Epub 2005 Jun 13.
39. Linderholm BK, Lindh B, Beckman L, Erlanson M, Edin K, Travelin B, Bergh J, Grankvist K, Henriksson R. Prognostic correlation of basic fibroblast growth factor and vascular endothelial growth factor in 1307 primary breast cancer. Clin Breast Cancer. 2003;4(5):340–7.
40. McCarthy NJ, Yang X, Linnoila IR, et al. Microvessel density, expression of estrogen receptor alpha, MIB-1, p53, and c-erbB-2 in inflammatory breast cancer. Clin Cancer Res. 2002;8:3857–62.
41. Miller KD, Chap LI, Holmes FA, Cobleigh MA, Marcom PK, Fehrenbacher L, Dickler M, Overmoyer BA, Reimann JD, Sing AP, Langmuir V, Rugo HS. Randomized phase III trial of capecitabine compared with bevacizumab plus capecitabine in

patients with previously treated metastatic breast cancer. J Clin Oncol. 2005;23(4):792–9.
42. Miller K, Wang M, Gralow J, Dickler M, Cobleigh M, Pérez EA, Shenkier T, Cella D, Davidson NE. Paclitaxel plus bevacizumab versus paclitaxel alone for metastatic breast cancer. N Engl J Med. 2007;357(26):2666–76.
43. Wedam SB, Low JA, Yang SX, et al. Antiangiogenic and antitumor effects of bevacizumab in patients with inflammatory and locally advanced breast cancer. J Clin Oncol. 2006;24:769–77.
44. Overmoyer B, Fu P, Hoppel C, et al. Inflammatory breast cancer as a model disease to study tumor angiogenesis: results of a phase IB trial of combination SU5416 and doxorubicin. Clin Cancer Res. 2007;13:5862–8.
45. Sonpavde G, Hutson TE. Pazopanib: a novel multitargeted tyrosine kinase inhibitor. Curr Oncol Rep. 2007;9:115–9.
46. Johnston SR, Hickish T, Ellis P, et al. Phase II study of the efficacy and tolerability of 2 dosing regimens of the farnesyl transferase inhibitor, R115777, in advanced breast cancer. J Clin Oncol. 2003;21:2492–9.

Follow-Up in Inflammatory Breast Cancer

11

Flavia Morales-Vasquez, Horacio Noe Lopez-Basave, and Martin Granados-Garcia

There are no changes in the guidelines that cite different treatment in the case of the follow-up of inflammatory breast cancer (IBC) and locally advanced breast cancer. Thus, treatment should adhere to the already established guidelines for locally advanced cancer of metastatic cancer of the breast.

Historically, it has been reported that on treating IBC with surgery alone or the combination of surgery plus radiotherapy (RT), mean survival is reported as <15 months, and local recurrence rates are reported as >50 % [1].

The result of treatment for IBC has improved impressively with the advent of multimodal treatment. Within a period of 20 years, with the introduction of anthracyclines, 5- and 10-year global survival (GS) rates of 40 % and 30 % have been reported, respectively [2, 3]. The incorporation of taxanes has been associated with better complete pathological response (cPR) rates and improvement in survival indices. According to the National Cancer Institute's Surveillance, Epidemiology and End Results (NCI SEER) database, between 1988 and 2001, mean 5-year survival was reported as 40 % for women with IBC against 87 % reported for all cases of breast cancer.

After recurrence, the majority of patients will die. Thus, IBC continues to be one of the most lethal forms of breast cancer.

In this chapter, our purpose is to define the term recurrence, to summarize the general recommendations, to describe the possible clinical condition, the risk factors, the treatment options, and their complications, and finally, in the conclusions, to highlight the focus toward which this treatment should be oriented.

Definition

Recurrent breast cancer is that which reappears after initial treatment when at least 6 months have elapsed without evidence of tumor activity after the patient has concluded the entire treatment.

Risk of recurrence is higher during the first 2 or 3 years after diagnosis, and this possibility diminishes continuously, although it will never reach zero, because there will always be the risk of recurrence in a patient who has presented this disease.

From 10 to 20 % of all recurrences are at the locoregional level, and 60–70 % will be metastases in one or multiple localizations. The

F. Morales-Vasquez, M.D., M.S. (✉)
Department of Medical Oncology, Instituto Nacional de Cancerologia-Mexico, San Fernando Num 22, Tlalpan, Mexico City, DF 14080, Mexico
e-mail: fabymvmizpah@aol.com

H.N. Lopez-Basave, M.S. • M. Granados-Garcia
Department of Oncological Surgery, Instituto Nacional de Cancerologia-Mexico, Mexico City, DF, Mexico

J.G. de la Garza-Salazar et al. (eds.), *Inflammatory Breast Cancer*,
DOI 10.1007/978-0-85729-991-8_11, © Springer-Verlag London 2013

Table 11.1 Recommendations for the follow-up of patients

Procedure	Frequency
Orientation of the patient on the signs and symptoms of recurrence	At the end of the patient's treatment
Physical examination by an oncologist or breast cancer specialist	Every 3 months for the first 2 years Every 6 months from years 3–5 Annually from year 5 on
Breast self-exploration	Monthly, rest of life
Mastography	Every 6 months for the first 2 years Annually from year 3
Tomographies, bone gammagram, hepatic enzymes	Only in the presence of symptoms
Tumor markers	Not recommended
Scrutiny for other neoplasms, such as endometrial, ovarian, or colon cancer	Annually

incidence and localization of the recurrence will depend on the initial tumor stage, the previous treatment, the tumor biology, and the sensitivity of the diagnosis [4, 5].

General Recommendations

Adequate Follow-Up After Treatment [6, 7]

The main objective of the follow-up of patients who have ended their adjuvant therapy or during this is being able to carry out early diagnosis of recurrent disease with the objective of the timely institution of adequate treatment. In Table 11.1, the following internationally accepted recommendations for the follow-up of these patients are described: orientation and education on the signs and symptoms of recurrence, self-exploration and periodic physical exploration by medical oncologists, and studies including mastography, ultrasound (US), and the pertinent laboratory studies and their periodicity.

Table 11.2 Studies that are not recommended in routine fashion

Studies that are not recommended in asymptomatic patients
Tumor markers
Chest wall x-rays
Thoracic and abdominal tomographies
Bone tracking
PET (positron emission tomography)

There are without doubt many more diagnostic resources; however, they are of dubious value for timely diagnosis because the appearance of metastases after primary treatment is alien to the physician, and the imaging or laboratory studies in themselves do not anticipate the diagnosis of recurrence. At this time and in the light of the literature and the different international consensuses, first intention tumor markers, chest wall x-rays, tomographies, nuclear medicine studies, or positron-emission tomography-computed tomography (PET-CT) are not recommended, except in specific situations and in a secondary manner (see Table 11.2).

Identify the Expression of Hormone Receptors and HER2 [8]

In the case of documenting the recurrence, it is necessary to identify again in the biopsy of the recurrent tissue the status of the hormone receptors estrogen, progesterone, and HER2 due to the possibility that changes in their expression are very frequent and knowledge of these allows offering a better treatment.

Restaging

Meticulous physical exploration and restaging by means of laboratory and imaging studies according to the findings of the exploration and the presenting signs and symptoms are necessary. In some series of postmortem examinations in patients with breast cancer [9, 10], the most frequent sites of metastasis are bone, liver, lung, and locoregional-level disease (see Table 11.3).

Table 11.3 Breast cancer metastases

Localization	Clinical findings (%)	Findings on necropsy (%)
CNS	5–10	30–50
Lung/pleura	15–20	50–75
Local/locoregional heart	20–40	30–50
Heart	<5	25–40
Liver	5–15	50–75
Bone	20–60	60–90
Intra-abdominal	<5	30–40
Ovary	<5	20–40

CNS central nervous system

Classification of Local or Disseminated Disease [10]

As soon as recurrence has been documented and a careful assessment has been made on the extension of the disease, the recurrence should be divided into locoregional or distant but resectable against unresectable disseminated disease because in the first situation, treatment should be carried out with a curative intent and surgery can comprise the cornerstone of this.

Establishment of the Scope of the Treatment [11]

In metastatic breast cancer, the treatment objectives intend to:

- Prolong the progression-free interval (PFI) and global survival (GS)
- Palliate the symptoms
- Maintain adequate quality of life (QoL) with good functional state

Selection of the Best Therapeutic Strategy [12–14]

To achieve these objectives, the best therapeutic strategy should be chosen, taking into account the tumor biology and the clinical factors, thus determining the most adequate treatment for each patient in particular [12–14].

These include:

- Age
- Symptoms
- Functional state
- Concomitant diseases
- Disease-free interval (DFI)
- Aggressiveness of the disease
- Site, number, and volume of the metastases
- Prior treatment and response to same
- Patient's preference
- Hormone receptors and HER2 overexpression-amplification

All patients with metastatic disease should receive systemic treatment according to their characteristics.

Clinical Condition, Risk Factors, Treatment Options, and Their Complications

The most important issue in terms of defining the clinical condition will be determined by the disease site of the recurrence, concerning which it is relevant to define whether the recurrence is local, locoregional, distant at a unique site, or distant at multiple sites.

Local Recurrence

Local recurrence is generally treated in a curative manner [4, 6]. There always exists the difficulty of distinguishing between a locoregional recurrence and a second ipsilateral neoplasm. The characteristics that can suggest a second neoplasm to us are the following:

- Prolonged disease-free period from the date of diagnosis of the first tumor and the appearance of the second tumor in the breast
- Different localization in the breast
- Tumor with different biological characteristics, such as histology, grade of differentiation, different expression of hormone receptors, as well as of HER2

Five-year GS in an isolated chest wall recurrence is 68 % against 81 % at the breast site [1].

In the case of being operable, all unique-, local-, regional-, or isolated-site recurrence should be resected, offering neoplasm-free surgical margins.

The net benefit of surgical treatment is clearly greater in recurrent disease with unique-site activity, but confusing when the recurrence is accompanied by metastasis at several sites, especially visceral.

Similarly, the impact of surgical treatment on GS has not been evaluated in a consistent manner. When the recurrence is in a conservative surgically treated breast and to the extent possible, continue with conservative surgical management of the breast.

The definition of local or locoregional recurrence includes recurrence in the breast after conservative breast surgery, recurrence in chest wall after mastectomy, recurrence in supra- and infraclavicular, parasternal, or ipsilateral lymph nodes, and in the skin of the chest wall and/or in that of the reconstructed breast.

With respect to the approach to this recurrence, surgery is available, which will be first choice in the case of ensuring adequate surgical margins and preferably without other disease sites.

Radiotherapy, whether in adjuvant form or as a palliative resource, is a means that is available for the management of recurrent disease, especially at the level of the bone, of the upper nervous system, and in some situations at the locoregional level, where superficial treatment of the inflammatory-type cutaneous disease can be offered.

Systemic treatment will be similar to that which is available and is usually indicated for metastatic breast cancer (see Table 11.4).

Considering the heterogeneity of recurrent or metastatic breast cancer, it is clear that this can present with different factors of greater or lesser aggressivity, which should be taken into account for selecting the best treatment in each particular case.

The scoring of the risk is traditionally based on the expression of hormone receptors, overexpression of HER2, the disease-free period, the amount of sites affected by the disease, whether there is visceral affectation or not, and whether or not there is vital organ involvement (see Table 11.5).

Table 11.4 Treatment options for patients with recurrent breast cancer at the local and systemic level

Hormonal therapy (tamoxifen, aromatase inhibitors, fulvestrant, GnRH analogs)
Chemotherapy (anthracyclines, taxanes, capecitabine, vinorelbine, etc.)
Therapy with monoclonal antibodies (trastuzumab, bevacizumab)
Tyrosine kinase inhibitors (lapatinib)
Biphosphonates
Radiotherapy
Ablative/palliative surgical procedures
Combined/sequential treatments
Other procedures, such as pleurodesis, laparoscopic surgery, ablations

Table 11.5 Risk evaluation

Low	Characteristics	High
Yes	Presence of hormone receptors	No
No	Overexpression of HER 2	Yes
>2 years	Disease-free interval	<2 years
Limited	Number of metastases	Extensive
Soft tissues and bone	Site of the metastasis	Visceral
No	Involvement of vital organs	Yes

Treatment According to Risk

Patients with low risk are usually hormonosensitive, and an attempt should be made to treat them initially with hormone therapy. Contrariwise, those at high risk should initiate treatment with chemotherapy.

(a) Characteristics of patients who are candidates for initial management with hormone therapy:
   Patients who are candidates for hormone therapy should have tumors that present:
   Hormone receptors that are both positive (requisite condition)

Prolonged DFS (2 years or more)
Metastasis in soft tissues and/or in bone
With metastatic disease of slow evolution

(b) Characteristics of patients who are candidates for initial treatment with chemotherapy:
Patients with tumors that present HER2 +++ (or fluorescent in situ hybridization [FISH]+)
Negative hormone receptors
Hormone-resistant tumors
DFI of <12 months
Presence of visceral metastases
Symptoms requiring a rapid palliative response

Hormone Therapy

Management with hormone therapy when indicated, that is, prior to the expression of hormonal receptors and scarcely symptomatic disease, will depend on the menstrual status.

The following criteria allow definition of menopause [15]:

Age ≥60 years

Age <60 years with amenorrhea of 12 months not associated with chemotherapy/hormone therapy (CT/HT) with follicle-stimulating hormone (FSH) and estradiol at postmenopausal levels.

In the case of chemotherapy-induced menopause, verification of the hormone state by means of estrogen quantification (estrogens <50 pg/ml; estradiol <30 pg/ml). This measure should be repeated to corroborate the menstrual state at 6 and at 12 months.

Hormone Treatment in Premenopausal Women

Tamoxifen is the first-line treatment of choice in patients without prior hormone therapy. In case of progression to tamoxifen but with initial objective response to tamoxifen or when patients have received adjuvant therapy prior to this drug, ovarian ablation (surgical or chemical) will be indicated, to be accompanied by aromatase inhibitors whenever possible [16–18]. At present, fulvestrant is also available as third-line hormone therapy.

Hormone Treatment in Postmenopausal Women

When first-line treatment with tamoxifen or aromatase inhibitors is recommended, selection will depend on drug availability and the comorbilities of the patients; in the case of having utilized tamoxifen previously, the second-line treatment indicated is aromatase inhibitors [19–24]. If the patients received tamoxifen and nonsteroidal aromatase inhibitors (anastrozole or letrozole), an additional treatment option that can be considered is steroidal aromatase inhibitors (exemestane) [25] and a pure antiestrogen (fulvestrant) [26, 27].

In patients with response or with clear clinical benefit with hormone therapy and who progress to a first-line therapy, an attempt should be made with a second- or third-line hormone therapy, depending on which was utilized previously, because a new tumor response is frequently obtained [22, 23]. In the case of resistance to hormone management, chemotherapy should be attempted.

Finally, the possibility should be considered of employing an aromatase inhibitor plus trastuzumab or lapatinib in patients with positive hormone receptors and HER2-positive receptors whenever chemotherapy is contraindicated [28]. In the case of patients with high risk but with positive receptors who have received chemotherapy up to the maximum benefit, these should receive hormone therapy according to their menstrual status and to the availability of the drugs.

Chemotherapy and Target Therapies in Recurrent Breast Cancer

These patients are classified into three groups:

(a) HER2-negative or unknown
(b) HER2-positive (immunohistochemistry +++ or FISH-positive)
(c) Triple-negative (estrogen receptors, progesterone receptors, and HER2-negatives)

Table 11.6 Recommendations for treatment with chemotherapy

Prior treatment	None or without anthracyclines	With anthracyclines	With anthracyclines and taxanes
First-line	Based on anthracyclines	Taxanes ± Capecitabine a Gemcitabine[a]	Capecitabine[b] Gemcitabine[b]

[a]Evidence level 2a
[b]Depending on first-line ± anti-Her2 therapy

Systemic treatment in patients with HER2-negative or unknown (75–80 % of cases)

1. First-line Systemic Treatment
   There is no standard first-line management regimen for patients with metastatic, HER2-negative, nonhormonosensitive breast cancer. Several considerations will be taken into account to choose the best treatment, with important points comprising the prior adjuvant treatment (see Table 11.6) and the interval of the end of the adjuvancy (greater or lesser than 1 year) because in patients who relapse after 1 year, first-line treatment could include drugs administered in adjuvancy. In patients with important symptoms and/or rapidly progressing visceral metastases, the therapy of choice is the combination based on higher response percentages and rapid palliation. Which combination will be chosen? This will depend on the patients' characteristics, their comorbilities, symptoms to be palliated, and the availability of drugs. The cornerstone of first-line treatment are schemes with anthracyclines [26–28]. However, a high percentage of patients will have already received these with adjuvancy; thus, there are three approved schemes for these patients: two of these produce better GS and PFI (docetaxel/capecitabine and paclitaxel/gemcitabine) compared with taxane alone [29–31], and the third combination with bevacizumab plus paclitaxel or docetaxel only prolonged the PFI compared with taxane monotherapy [32–34]. If, contrariwise, there are no important symptoms to palliate, no nonvisceral disease or of slow evolution, the sequential treatment can be selected, initiating with monotherapy (taxane) [35–37] or capecitabine (patients who received the taxane with adjuvancy) [37]. The combination with capecitabine and docetaxel compared with docetaxel alone, after failure with anthracyclines, produces a total response (TR) percentage of 42 versus 30 %, total survival (TS) of 14.5 versus 11.5 months, with a time of progression of 6.1 versus 4.2 months, but superior toxicity for combined schemes with grades III–IV diarrhea of 62 versus 42 %, stomatitis of 65 versus 40 %, and hand-foot syndrome of 65 versus 7 %.

   Treatment duration has not been well defined [38]; the time will depend on the drug that is being applied (i.v. vs. oral, maximum accumulated doses), the toxicity, and the patient's QoL.

   Treatment with chemotherapy in the metastatic disease scenario should be carried out as soon as equilibrium is achieved among tolerance, efficacy, and QoL.
2. In the case of HER2-positive (immunohistochemistry +++ or FISH-positive) patients, which constitutes 20 % of patients.
   Patients with overexpression of HER2 +++ by immunohistochemistry or fluorescent in situ hybridization (FISH)

   FISH+ (around 20–30 % of breast carcinomas) comprise a subgroup with poor prognosis and a greater probability of relapse. The employment of trastuzumab for 1 year in combination with chemotherapy in this group of patients achieves a diminution in risk of disease recurrence in approximately 50 % and in the risk of death in 30 %.

Within the context of already occurring recurrent disease, if there has been no prior treatment with trastuzumab, the latter should be offered with chemotherapy; in the case of prior adjuvant treatment with trastuzumab, this can be reinitiated in combination with chemotherapy. However, if there is progression with this combination, treatment can be continued with lapatinib, according to FDA approval for trastuzumab-resistant metastatic disease management. In theory and in some phase III studies, the combination of trastuzumab plus lapatinib with or without chemotherapy in HER2 disease has been tested.

Patients who receive trastuzumab should be carefully assessed due to the risk of cardiotoxicity, especially those with a personal history of cardiac disease of who are at high risk. All patients who receive this drug should be monitored by means of echocardiography (ECHO) for timely detection of diminution in ventricular function.

The Triple-Negative Patient (Estrogen Receptors, Progesterone Receptors, and HER2-Negative)

This group of women with breast cancer is related with poor prognosis, in whom antihormone therapy and epidermal growth factor (EGF)-directed antibodies are not useful. The unique treatment option for these patients is chemotherapy.

Chemotherapy for this group of patients continues to be the established treatment for metastatic breast disease. There are data in small phase II studies that suggest that some agents could offer a greater benefit, such as platinum salts and alkylating agents, and in the case of *BRCA 1* and *BRCA 2* genetic alterations, poly ADP ribose polymerase enzyme (PARP) inhibitors could be of great benefit; however, there are no modifications in the specific treatment regimens for this group of patients.

At present, there are treatments against novel molecular targets that are under study, such as the vascular endothelial growth factor (VEGF), with a study of paclitaxel plus bevacizumab for metastatic disease. An increase is shown in GS; however, although this strategy is approved by the US Federal Drug Administration (FDA), it cannot be recommended in Mexico except in a clinical study.

Anthracycline- and Taxane-Resistant Recurrent Breast Cancer

These are patients who have been treated previously in adjuvant form, or patients with measurable disease who present disease recurrence within a period of <1 year, or patients in whom evident disease progression is observed during treatment with these agents.

Under these circumstances, the drugs available to continue treatment in measurable disease are:

Cytotoxics:
- Gemcitabine
- Capecitabine
- Vinorelbine
- Pegylated adriamycin
- Ixabepilone

Biological agents:
- Trastuzumab
- Lapatinib
- Bevacizumab

The efficiency of each of these has been proven, identifying an average response of 30 % in general for all of these. The disease is recognized as a noncurable clinical condition; thus, the toxicity that will be provided should be assessed. Evaluation of when combinations (doublets) are employed has been achieved, in which it is possible to reach a slight increase in the response level of approximately 35–44 %, but this at the cost of the nearly double toxicity of chemotherapy schemes involving a sole agent or monodrug.

In patients with resistance to anthracyclines and taxanes but with HER2 (+), it is possible to continue anti-HER2 treatment with trastuzumab or lapatinib in those who failed with adriamycin and taxanes; a phase III study with a dose of capecitabine 1,250 mg 1–14 plus trastuzumab showed global response (GR) in 45 %, complete response (CR) in 15 %, partial response (PR) in 30 %, and stable disease in 33 %. Mean survival was 28 months and disease-free survival (DFS) was 6.7 months. The safety profile includes predictable toxicity [39, 40].

Another scheme employed in the HER2 (+) group that failed with anthracyclines and taxanes is vinorelbine + trastuzumab in a phase II study with 54 patients and an overall response (OR) of 66 %, but this percentage of response has not been demonstrated in any phase III study. Checking the left ventricle ejection fraction (LVEF) is recommended every 16 months as cardiac monitoring [41].

In anthracycline- and taxane-resistant breast cancer, the combination of ixabepilone and capecitabine was superior to capecitabine alone. A phase III study with 752 patients showed an increase in objective response (35 vs. 14 %) and an increase in the PFI of 5.8 versus 4.2 months [42].

A phase II study compared albumin-bound paclitaxel versus polyethoxylated castor oil-based paclitaxel, with 454 patients, of whom 66 % with failure to anthracyclines. The former paclitaxel treatment does not require premedication. There was a mean time to progression of 31 versus 22 weeks, respectively, and TS of 56.4 versus 46.7 months [43].

Another phase II study comparing vinorelbine with monodrug 30 mg/m^2 versus vinorebine + gemcitabine 1,200 mg/m^2 for 1–8/21 days showed a mean survival to progression of 4 versus 6 months, TS of 16.4 versus 15.9 months, and toxicity III–III, 44 versus 61 % [44].

Treatment of Recurrent Breast Cancer in Elderly Patients

This group of patients is more and more frequent in Mexico, due to the aging of the population. *There is evidence that the disease at this age is less aggressive because in general it corresponds to tumors with a low proliferation rate, positive receptors, high frequency of diploidy, low expression of HER2, and low frequency of p53 mutation.* However, there is also an important group of patients with negative receptors or HER-positive receptors.

On the other hand, in this group of patients at an advanced age, functional state and concomitant diseases can render aggressive treatment difficult. Thus, it is recommended to *assess each case according to validated geriatric scales in oncological patients, including ADL (activities of daily living) or CGA (comprehensive geriatric assessment)*:

(a) Hormone treatment is recommended for patients with RH+.
(b) In patients who are RH-negative or hormone therapy-resistant, chemotherapy is recommended, based on monodrug schemes and not on chemotherapy schemes in which two or three agents are combined.
(c) In this palliative scenario, it should not be forgotten that quality of life is fundamental.
(d) In patients with HER2+, the possible benefit will be assessed of trastuzumab, taking its eventual cardiotoxicity into consideration.

Role of Biphosphonates in the Prevention of Breast Cancer Recurrence

The biphosphonates constitute standard management for metastatic bone disease, bone-metastases-induced hypercalcemia, as well as for the prevention of bone mineral density loss. It has even been documented that with the monthly i.v. application of zoledronic acid, an increase is achieved in the GS of some patients with metastatic bone disease [45, 46].

Recently, a promising reduction has been cited of breast cancer recurrence, thanks to the employment of biphosphonates. Four early studies with clodronate demonstrated the potential of biphosphonates in preventing bone metastases and prolonging survival; however, results have not been consistent. Recently, the most active biphosphonate, zoledronic acid, administered i.v. every

6 months, demonstrated prevention of bone mineral loss and the reduction of the risk of bone events in 36 % ($p = 0.01$) compared with adjuvant treatment based on hormone therapy alone, in the Zometa-Femara Adjuvant Synergy Trial (ZO-FAST) [47–52].

Thus, diverse clinical assays are found to be considering different biphosphonates, and it is necessary to evaluate the results to determine the real impact on the increase in GS and above all the prevention that there could be in terms of recurrent disease.

Treatment Duration

Optimal duration of therapy with bisphosphonates is not well defined. The recommendation is as follows [53]:

- Treatment with diphosphonates during 2 years and after this, reconsideration of its use.
- The considerations can comprise still active cancer and existing foci of metastasis.
- If the treatment is discontinued, initiate strict surveillance.

Treatment Complications

These can be acute influenza syndrome 15–30 %, renal complications, above all in rapid intravenous (i.v.) infusions with high doses, osteonecrosis of the jaw, above all, associated with dental extractions and infections. The following is recommended:

- Oral examination every 6–12 months and avoidance of dental surgery unless there is no other alternative
- Blood chemistry prior to each application
- Contraindicated in creatinine depuration of <30 ml/min

References

1. Zucali R, Uslenghi C, Kenda R, Bonadonna G. Natural history and survival of inoperable breast cancer treated with radiotherapy and radiotherapy followed by radical mastectomy. Cancer. 1976;37(3):1422–31.
2. Ueno NT, Buzdar AU, Singletary SE, Ames FC, McNeese MD, Holmes FA, Theriault RL, Strom EA, Wasaff BJ, Asmar L, Frye D, Hortobagyi GN. Combined-modality treatment of inflammatory breast carcinoma: twenty years of experience at MD Anderson Cancer Center. Cancer Chemother Pharmacol. 1997;40(4):321–9.
3. Hortobagyi GN, de la Garza Salazar J, Pritchard K, Amadori D, Haidinger R, Hudis CA, Khaled H, Liu MC, Martin M, Namer M, O'Shaughnessy JA, Shen ZZ, Albain KS, ABREAST Investigators. The global breast cancer burden: variations in epidemiology and survival (review). Clin Breast Cancer. 2005;6(5):391–401.
4. Yoshida T, Takei H, Kurosumi M, Ninomiya J, Ishikawa Y, Hayashi Y, Tozuka K, Oba H, Kawanowa K, Inoue K, Tabei T. True recurrences and new primary tumors have different clinical features in invasive breast cancer patients with ipsilateral breast tumor relapse after breast-conserving treatment. Breast J. 2010;16(2):127–33. Epub 2009 Dec 21.
5. Huber KE, Carey LA, Wazer DE. Breast cancer molecular subtypes in patients with locally advanced disease: impact on prognosis, patterns of recurrence, and response to therapy (review). Semin Radiat Oncol. 2009;19(4):204–10.
6. Segunda Revisión del Consenso Nacional sobre el diagnóstico y tratamiento del Cáncer mamario. Colima; 2005.
7. NCCN (National Comprehensive Cancer Network). NCCN practice guidelines in oncology: breast cancer. 2012. Available at: http://www.nccn.org/professionals/physician_gls/pdf/breast.pdf. Mar 2012.
8. López-Guerrero JA, Llombart-Cussac A, Noguera R, Navarro S, Pellin A, Almenar S, Vázquez-Alvadalejo C, Llombart-Bosch A. HER2 amplification in recurrent breast cancer following breast-conserving therapy correlates with distant metastasis and poor survival. Int J Cancer. 2006;118(7):1743–9.
9. Rhee J, Han SW, Oh DY, et al. The clinicopathologic characteristics and prognostic significance of triple-negativity in node-negative breast cancer. BMC Cancer. 2008;8:307.
10. Kamby C, Ejlertsen B, Andersen J, et al. The pattern of metastases in human breast cancer. Influence of systemic adjuvant therapy and impact on survival. Acta Oncol. 1988;27:715–9.
11. Early Breast Cancer Trialists' Collaborative Group. Effects of chemotherapy and hormonal therapy in breast cancer on recurrence and 15-year survival: an overview of the randomized trials. Lancet. 2005;365: 1687–717.
12. Giordano SH, Buzdar AU, Smith TL, et al. Is breast cancer survival improving? Cancer. 2004;100:44.
13. Gennari A, Conte P, Rosso R, et al. Survival of metastatic breast carcinoma patients over a 20-year period. Cancer. 2005;104:1742.
14. González-Angulo AM, Morales-Vásquez F, Hortobagyi GN. Overview of resistance to systemic therapy in patients with breast cancer (review). Adv Exp Med Biol. 2007;608:122.
15. Soules MR, Sherman S, Parrott E, Rebar R. Executive summary: stages of reproductive aging workshop (STRAW). Fertil Steril. 2001;76:874.

16. Nabholtz JM, Buzdar A, Pollak M, et al. Anastrozole is superior to tamoxifen as first-line therapy for advanced breast carcinoma is postmenopausal women: results of a North America multicenter randomized trial. J Clin Oncol. 2000;18:3758–67.
17. Bonaterre J, Thurlimann B, Robertson JFR, et al. Anastrozole versus tamoxifen as first-line therapy for advanced breast cancer in 668 postmenopausal women: results of the Tamoxifen or Arimidex Randomized Group Efficacy and Tolerability Study. J Clin Oncol. 2000;18:3748–57.
18. Mouridsen H, Gersanovich M, Sun Y, et al. Phase III study of letrozole versus tamoxifen as first-line therapy of advanced breast cancer in postmenopausal women: analysis of survival and update of efficacy from the International Letrozole Breast Cancer Group. J Clin Oncol. 2003;21:2101–9.
19. Lonning PE, Bajetta E, Murray R, et al. Activity of exemestane in metastatic breast cancer after failure of nonsteroidal aromatase inhibitors: a phase II trials. J Clin Oncol. 2000;18:2234–44.
20. Watanabe T, Sano M, Ohno S, et al. Fulvestrant for the treatment of advanced breast cancer in postmenopausal women: a Japanese study. Anticancer Res. 2004;24:1275.
21. Howell A, Pippen J, Elledge RM, et al. Fulvestrant versus anastrozole for the treatment of advanced breast carcinoma. Cancer. 2005;104:236.
22. Osborne CK, Pippen J, Jones SE, et al. Double-blind, randomized trial comparing the efficacy and tolerability of fulvestrant versus anastrozole in postmenopausal women with advanced breast cancer progressing on prior endocrine therapy: results of a North American trial. J Clin Oncol. 2002;20:3386.
23. Howell A, Robertson JF, Quaresma Albano J, et al. Fulvestrant, formerly ICI 182,780, is as effective as anastrozole in postmenopausal women with advanced breast cancer progressing after prior endocrine treatment. J Clin Oncol. 2002;20:3396.
24. Ingle JN, Suman VJ, Rowland KM, et al. Fulvestrant in women with advanced breast cancer after progression on prior aromatase inhibitor therapy: North Central Cancer Treatment Group Trial N0032. J Clin Oncol. 2006;24:1052.
25. Chia S, Gradishar W, Mauriac L, et al. Double-blind, randomized placebo controlled trial of fulvestrant compared with exemestane after prior nonsteroidal aromatase inhibitor therapy in postmenopausal women with hormone receptor-positive, advanced breast cancer: results from EFECT. J Clin Oncol. 2008;26:1664.
26. Johnston SJ, Cheung KL. Fulvestrant- a novel endocrine therapy for breast cancer (review). Curr Med Chem. 2010;17(10):902–14.
27. Robertson JF, Llombart-Cussac A, Rolski J, Feltl D, Dewar J, Macpherson E, Lindemann J, Ellis MJ. Activity of fulvestrant 500 mg versus anastrozole 1mg as first-line treatment for advanced breast cancer: results from the FIRST study. J Clin Oncol. 2009;27(27):4530–5. Epub 2009 Aug 24.
28. Johnston S, Pergram M, Press M, et al. Lapatinib combined with letrozole vs. letrozole alone for front line postmenopausal hormone receptor positive (HR+) metastatic breast cancer (MBC). J Clin Oncol. 2009;27:5538–46.
29. Hortobagyi GN, Yap HY, Kau SW, et al. A comparative study of doxorubicin and epirubicin in patients with metastatic breast cancer. Am J Clin Oncol. 1989; 12:57.
30. Falkson G, Tormey DC, Carey P, et al. Long-term survival of patients treated with combination chemotherapy for metastatic breast cancer. Eur J Cancer. 1991;27:973.
31. Hortobagyi GN, Bodey GP, Buzdar AU, et al. Evaluation of high-dose versus standard FAC chemotherapy for advanced breast cancer in protected environment units: a prospective randomized study. J Clin Oncol. 1987;5:354.
32. Conte PF, Guarneri V, Bruzzi P, et al. Concomitant versus sequential administration of epirubicin and paclitaxel as first-line therapy in metastatic breast carcinoma: results for the Gruppo Oncologico Nord Ovest randomized trial. Cancer. 2004;101:704.
33. O'Shaughnessy J, et al. Superior survival with capecitabine plus docetaxel. Combination therapy in anthracycline-pretreatment patients with advanced breast cancer. Phase III trial result. J Clin Oncol. 2002;12:2812–23.
34. Carrick S, Parker S, Wilcken N, et al. Single agent versus combination chemotherapy for metastatic breast cancer. Cochrane Database Syst Rev. 2005:CD003372.
35. Blum JL, Dieras V, Lo Russo PM, et al. Multicenter, phase II study of capecitabine in taxane-pretreated metastatic breast carcinoma patients. Cancer. 2001;92:1759.
36. Fumoleau P, Largillier R, Clippe C, et al. Multicentre, phase II study evaluating capecitabine monotherapy in patients with anthracycline- and taxane-pretreated metastatic breast cancer. Eur J Cancer. 2004;40: 536.
37. Reichardt P, Von Minckwitz G, Thuss-Patience PC, et al. Multicenter phase II study of oral capecitabine (Xeloda)in patients with metastatic breast cancer relapsing after treatment with a taxane-containing therapy. Ann Oncol. 2003;14:1227.
38. Gennari A, D'amico M, Corradengo D. Extending the duration of first-line chemotherapy in metastatic breast cancer: a perspective review. Ther Adv Med Oncol. 2011;3(5):229–232. doi:10.1177/1758834011413423
39. O'Shaughnessy J, Twelves C, Aapro M. Treatment for anthracycline-pretreated metastatic breast cancer. (Review). Oncologist. 2002;7 Suppl 6:4–12.
40. Schaller G, Fuchs I, Gonsch T, Weber J, Kleine-Tebbe A, Klare P, Hindenburg HJ, Lakner V, Hinke A, Bangemann N. Phase II study of capecitabine plus

trastuzumab in human epidermal growth factor receptor 2 overexpressing metastatic breast cancer pretreated with anthracyclines or taxanes. J Clin Oncol. 2007;25(22):3246–50. Epub 2007 Jun 18.
41. Burstein HJ, Harris LN, Marcom PK, Lambert-Falls R, Havlin K, Overmoyer B, Friedlander Jr RJ, Gargiulo J, Strenger R, Vogel CL, Ryan PD, Ellis MJ, Nunes RA, Bunnell CA, Campos SM, Hallor M, Gelman R, Winer EP. Trastuzumab and vinorelbine as first-line therapy for HER2-overexpressing metastatic breast cancer: multicenter phase II trial with clinical outcomes, analysis of serum tumor markers as predictive factors, and cardiac surveillance algorithm. J Clin Oncol. 2003;21(15):2889–95.
42. Thomas ES, Gómez HL, Li RK, Chung HC, Fein LE, Chan VF, Jassem J, Pivot XB, Klimovsky JV, de Mendoza FH, Xu B, Campone M, Lerzo GL, Peck RA, Mukhopadhyay P, Vahdat LT, Roché HH. Ixabepilone plus capecitabine for metastatic breast cancer progressing after anthracycline and taxane treatment. J Clin Oncol. 2007;25(33):5210–7. Epub 2007 Oct 29.
43. Gradishar WJ, Tjulandin S, Davidson N, Shaw H, Desai N, Bhar P, Hawkins M, O'Shaughnessy J. Phase III trial of nanoparticle albumin-bound paclitaxel compared with polyethylated castor oil-based paclitaxel in women with breast cancer. J Clin Oncol. 2005;23(31):7794–803. Epub 2005 Sep 19.
44. Martín M, Ruiz A, Muñoz M, Balil A, García-Mata J, Calvo L, Carrasco E, Mahillo E, Casado A, García-Sáenz JA, Escudero MJ, Guillem V, Jara C, Ribelles N, Salas F, Soto C, Morales-Vásquez F, Rodríguez CA, Adrover E, Mel JR, Spanish Breast Cancer Research Group (GEICAM) trial. Gemcitabine plus vinorelbine versus vinorelbine monotherapy in patients with metastatic breast cancer previously treated with anthracyclines and taxanes: final results of the phase III Spanish Breast Cancer Research Group (GEICAM) trial. Lancet Oncol. 2007;8(3):219–25.
45. Coleman RE. Bisphosphonates in breast cancer. Ann Oncol. 2005;16:687–95.
46. Winter MC, Coleman RE. Bisphosphonates in breast cancer: teaching an old dog new tricks. Curr Opin Oncol. 2009;21:499–506.
47. Coleman WY. Meta-analysis of clodronate and breast cancer survival. Br J Cancer. 2007;96:1796–801.
48. Coleman RE. Adjuvant bisphosphonates in breast cancer: Are we witnessing the emergence of a new tHER 2apeutic strategy? Eur J Cancer. 2009. doi:10.1016/j.
49. Eidtmann H, Bundred NJ, DeBoer R. The effect of zoledronic acid on aromatase inhibitor associated bone loss in postmenopausal women with early breast cancer receiving adjuvant letrozole: 36 months follow-up of ZO-FAST. Cancer Res. 2008;69(Suppl 2). Abstract 44. San Antonio breast cancer symposium.
50. Gnant M, Mlineritsch B, Schippinger W, et al. Endocrine tHER 2apy plus zoledronic acid in premenopausal breast cancer. N Engl J Med. 2009;360(7): 679–91.
51. Pavlakis N, Schmidt R, Stockler M. Bisphosphonates for breast cancer. Cochrane Database Syst Rev 2005;(3):CD003474. Epub 2005 Jul 20.
52. Rosen LS, Gordon DH, et al. Zoledronic acid is superior to pamidronate for the treatment of bone metastases in breast carcinoma patients with at least one osteolytic lesion. Cancer. 2004;100:36–43.
53. NCCN Task Force Report. Bone health in cancer care. J Natl Compr Canc Netw. 2009;7 Suppl 3:1–32.

Index

J.G. de la Garza-Salazar et al. (eds.), *Inflammatory Breast Cancer*,
DOI 10.1007/978-0-85729-991-8, © Springer-Verlag London 2013